<u>Heart Rhythms</u>

ALSO BY JEFFREY ROTHFEDER

Minds Over Matter:
A New Look at Artificial Intelligence

Heart Rhythms

By Jeffrey Rothfeder

Foreword by Jeremy N. Ruskin, M.D.
Introduction by J. Thomas Bigger, M.D.

LITTLE, BROWN AND COMPANY
BOSTON / TORONTO / LONDON

FIRST EDITION

Paul Dudley White's letter "The Tight Girdle Syndrome" is reprinted from *The New England Journal of Medicine* (Volume 288, p. 584). Copyright © 1973 Massachusetts Medical Society.

Credits:
The Way the Heart Works: The American Heart Association
Figure 1 and Figure 2: Leonard D. Dank/ Medical Illustrations Company

LIBRARY OF CONGRESS CATALOGING-IN-PUBLICATION DATA

Rothfeder, Jeffrey.
    Heart rhythms: breakthrough treatments that cure cardiac arrhythmia, the silent killer of 400,000 Americans each year / by Jeffrey Rothfeder; with a foreword by Jeremy Ruskin and an introduction by Thomas Bigger. — 1st ed.
        p.   cm.
    Includes index.
    ISBN 0-316-75785-3
    1. Arrhythmia — Popular works. I. Title.
RC685.A65R67 1988
616.1'2806 — dc 19   88-13251
                                                       CIP

10 9 8 7 6 5 4 3 2 1

FG

DESIGNED BY JEANNE ABBOUD

*Published simultaneously in Canada
by Little, Brown & Company (Canada) Limited*

PRINTED IN THE UNITED STATES OF AMERICA

To Hugh J. "Mac" MacDonald
(1925–1988),
the strongest man
I have ever known

Contents

Foreword

SUDDEN death due to arrhythmias accounts for approximately two-thirds of the 600,000 deaths annually that are attributable to cardiac disease in the United States. Most of these deaths, which result from electrical malfunctions of the heart known as arrhythmias, are instantaneous, occurring within seconds or minutes. And despite the fact that sudden cardiac death from arrhythmias kills more males in industrialized countries than any other condition, it remains one of the least understood and least publicized diseases in the world today.

Because of these disturbing statistics, the past decade has witnessed an explosion of research and clinical activity in the field of electrophysiology, the subspecialty of cardiology that deals with the electrical system of the heart and the abnormal rhythms that cause sudden death. New and important insights into the normal and abnormal physiology of the heart's electrical system have been gained from these efforts. In addition to the scientific knowledge that has accrued, the growth of electrophysiology as a clinical discipline has resulted in the development of more objective and precise techniques for diagnosing and treating cardiac arrhythmias. Some of these advances include the use of techniques to artificially start and stop arrhythmias in a hospital laboratory in order to analyze the mechanism of the arrhythmia and to locate the region of the heart from which the arrhythmia arises; the use of computerized mapping techniques to track and display the movement of electricity through the heart; and the development of new treatments, including specialized surgical techniques and implantable devices that continuously monitor electrical activity in the heart and deliver a shock to terminate life-threatening arrhythmias whenever they occur. *Heart Rhythms* explores the field of cardiac electrophysiology and conveys in terms comprehensible to the nonmedical reader some of the important new concepts and techniques that are currently employed in the diagnosis and treatment of abnormal heart rhythms.

Jeremy N. Ruskin, M.D.
Director, Cardiac Arrhythmia Service
Massachusetts General Hospital
Boston, Massachusetts

Author's Note

F IVE years ago, when I was founding editor of *Medicine & Computer* magazine, a now defunct journal that reported on high-tech clinical achievements, a press release landed on my desk. It was one of hundreds that I routinely read each month, usually with skepticism because of their exaggerated claims about frequently mundane medical devices and accomplishments. But this one was compelling.

The release described the work of Dr. Jeremy Ruskin and his colleagues at the Cardiac Arrhythmia Service at Massachusetts General Hospital in Boston. It detailed techniques for offering renewed life to those previously doomed to imminent death from cardiac arrhythmias, "our most lethal disease."

At first blush, this smacked of pure medical hyperbole. How could anyone call arrhythmias our most lethal disease? That seemed implausible in that pre-AIDS era; nothing could be worse than coronary artery disease, cancer, and stroke, I thought.

Intrigued but skeptical, I investigated further. I called Ruskin, visited Massachusetts General Hospital, and read all the clinical materials I could find on cardiac arrhythmias. Gradually, the picture became more and more focused. And as I followed the story, the statistics were nothing less than mind-boggling.

I found out that little-publicized cardiac arrhythmias were actually responsible for over 400,000 sudden deaths each year in the United States alone, more than two-thirds of all deaths linked to heart disease; it kills more men in the western world than any other disease. This was a major public health problem, but few, it seemed — except arrhythmia victims and their families and friends — knew anything about a disease that took so many lives in this country.

Even more important than what I discovered about the disease, though, was what I found out about the clinical work of Ruskin and his colleagues at Massachusetts General and at other arrhythmia centers around the country. Quietly, these physicians were developing innovative, creative, state-of-the-art techniques to remove the death sentence that cardiac arrhythmia dangles over its victims. Indeed, the success rate of modern electrophysiologists in treating arrhythmias is remarkable. Only 10 percent of the critically ill patients that these electrophysiologists treat have another life-threatening arrhythmia within two years. Compare this to traditional approaches to the disease, in which close to 40 percent have a second arrhythmic episode within only one year; many of these episodes are fatal.

For me, this was a marvelous medical story that begged to be told: on the one hand, there was a devastating disease that had done its damage unchecked for too many years; on the other hand, suddenly there was a blossoming of clinical achievements to defeat the disease. I spent many hours interviewing electrophysiologists, discussing their work and arrhythmias in general, and the more we talked, the more attracted to the subject I became. *Heart Rhythms* is the result of this exploration.

All of this was reason enough for me to devote four years to putting on paper the story of cardiac arrhythmias. But an untimely and tragic coda occurred during the very days when

I was completing *Heart Rhythms,* which makes the subject even more irresistible to me. My father-in-law, Hugh J. "Mac" MacDonald, a sixty-two-year-old muscular carpenter, collapsed suddenly on the job, an apparent victim of a heart attack and arrhythmias. Just twenty-four hours later he was dead.

And as we watched the life slip away from Mac and listened to him describe the episodic, troubling arrhythmic pounding in his chest that was silent to our ears but that he was sure we heard, I realized just how damaging arrhythmias could be. I knew that if arrhythmias could suddenly fell a six-foot-two-inch giant of a man, they could defeat the strongest of us.

At the moment that Mac left this world behind, I became even more convinced of what originally spurred me to write this book: the electrophysiologists who are devoting their careers to combating life-threatening arrhythmias are performing a medical miracle. Because of the electrophysiologists, thousands of patients have been granted the unexpected second chance of renewed life, and finally there is a real chance that, with future breakthroughs, arrhythmias will claim fewer and fewer victims in the coming years.

Acknowledgments

HEART RHYTHMS could not have been completed without the generous time and assistance given to the project by many people. I owe a huge debt of gratitude to the electrophysiologists and their clinical colleagues throughout the United States who put up with my persistent requests for facts, anecdotes, statistics, case histories, research notes, and musings about arrhythmias. Thanks especially to Dr. Jeremy N. Ruskin at Massachusetts General Hospital in Boston; Dr. Michel Mirowski at Sinai Hospital in Baltimore; Dr. Enriqué Carter at the Office of Health Technology Assessment in Washington, D.C.; Dr. Gordon Moe, one of the forefathers of arrhythmia research; Dr. J. Thomas Bigger at Columbia-Presbyterian Hospital in New York City; Vincent Cucciero, Vice-President for Program and Facilities Development at Massachusetts General Hospital; Martin Bander, historian at Massachusetts General Hospital; Dr. Steven Geevas at Leland Hospital in Baltimore; Dr. John Smialek, Maryland Medical Examiner; Dr. Douglas Weaver at Harborview Medical Center in Seattle; Dr. Leonard Cobb at the University of Washington School of Medicine in

Seattle; Dr. Richard Crampton at the University of Virginia Medical Center in Charlottesville; Diana Rockwell, a critical care nurse at the University of Virginia Medical Center in Charlottesville; Dr. Richard Cohen at the Harvard-Massachusetts Institute of Technology Center for Biomedical Engineering in Cambridge; Dr. Raymond Ideker and Dr. William Smith at the Duke University Medical Center in North Carolina.

I am also especially grateful to the many arrhythmia victims who opened the doors of their personal lives to me, telling me the most intimate details of their case histories and permitting me to watch as they underwent anti-arrhythmia procedures in electrophysiology labs and operating rooms. I have granted all of these patients anonymity so as to minimize any invasion of their personal lives that *Heart Rhythms* might represent.

Thanks to two of the best people in publishing, my editor, Jennifer Josephy, and my agent, Dominick Abel, for understanding the importance of a book on cardiac arrhythmias.

And finally, thanks to my family — my wife, Dorie, and my children, Alexis and Ben. Dorie's support, indulgence, easy sense of humor, and love while I grew more compulsive, obsessed, and petulant as the deadlines for *Heart Rhythms* neared, can never be adequately repaid. They endear her to me more than ever. Alexis and Ben are nothing less than the sweetest of diversions.

Introduction

HEART RHYTHMS is a significant achievement because arrhythmias of the heart are complex and little understood by patients and their families, and by many physicians as well. This book provides a clear picture of the genesis of the rhythm disturbances that are related to sudden cardiac death and associated diseases. This information is imparted in a way that reveals the feelings of those who experience rhythm disturbances.

Over the past twenty-five years a new specialty has developed in cardiology, that of clinical cardiac electrophysiology, which is devoted to better understanding the electrical behavior of the heart in health and disease in order to better manage rhythm and conduction problems. Jeffrey Rothfeder makes it clear what electrophysiologists do and what they are like. Mr. Rothfeder's book is the first, to my knowledge, to give such insight into this new field. The view is personal and provides depth. Obviously, space and research limitations did not permit Mr. Rothfeder to cover the activities of every prominent electrophysiologist, but he offers a broad, yet intimate, portrait of the inner workings of this branch of cardiology.

From my perspective the most important achievement of *Heart Rhythms* is the information provided on the most critical public health problem facing Western civilization — sudden cardiac death. An American dies suddenly and unexpectedly every minute of every day, causing an incredible emotional and economic burden on society. Nearly all of these fatal events are due to a severe form of cardiac rhythm disturbance called ventricular fibrillation. About half the sudden deaths are associated with acute heart attacks, but half are not and represent electrical accidents, which usually occur in persons who have had heart attacks in the remote past. We have learned that sudden cardiac death need not be the end of the road; persons who are lucky enough to be resuscitated quickly from a cardiac arrest rarely have an immediate recurrence of the lethal rhythm and often survive to lead productive lives for many years thereafter.

It is important for the public to understand thoroughly the sudden cardiac death problem, because it must participate actively in the struggle to conquer sudden death. Ultimately, it will be conquered when basic research and public health policy make it possible to eradicate atherosclerosis, thus preventing heart attacks and the scarring of the heart that permits the fatal rhythm disturbances. Until this goal is reached, we need a multipronged attack on sudden cardiac death.

Community programs can save many cardiac arrest victims. The Seattle story (chapter 10) shows us how an urban community can work together with its city officials and physicians to salvage almost 1,000 lives per year from cardiac arrests that otherwise would have been sudden cardiac deaths. One out of three citizens in Seattle is capable of performing cardiopulmonary resuscitation, preserving life until definitive treatment arrives. Such community programs require commitment, donation of time, and high funding relative to competing projects. The Charlottesville experience (chapter 11) shows that a very different set of problems face rural communities, but these too can be solved to the benefit of the citizens.

Once a cardiac arrest victim has been salvaged, the electrophysiologist can nearly always find an effective method for preventing fatal recurrences. The methods used and the patients' experiences are starkly described in this book. It is unfortunate that patients must undergo a catastrophe in order to be referred to the help they need. Most of those who are vulnerable to cardiac arrest could be recognized by noninvasive testing, but widespread screening is very expensive. In the future, it is hoped, screening will be done on patients who have had attacks and on those from other high-risk groups to identify those most prone to future cardiac arrest, so that effective preventive treatment can be instituted.

Research and control programs can flourish only if there is widespread public knowledge of the sudden-death problem and approaches to its solution. Mr. Rothfeder has given us a human and fascinating insight into the area of rhythm and conduction disturbances of the heart and the men and women who combat these problems.

J. Thomas Bigger, M.D.
Director, Arrhythmia Control Unit
Columbia-Presbyterian Medical Center
New York, New York

Heart Rhythms

The Way the Heart Works

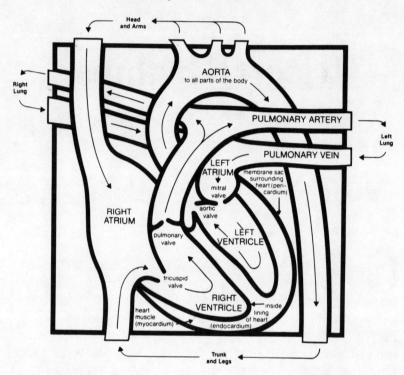

Right Heart
receives blood from
the body and pumps
it through the pul-
monary artery to the
lungs where it picks
up fresh oxygen.

Left Heart
receives oxygen-full
blood from the lungs
and pumps it
through the aorta to
the body

·1·

The Most Lethal Public Health Problem

IN 1982, for the first time in twenty years, Samuel W. took a long summer vacation, a fourteen-day unstructured August junket by the shore with his wife. It ended with the Labor Day weekend. For him, it was a necessary and much-deserved break. The sixty-two-year-old New York accountant was overworked and had been growing progressively more tired for months. He was burdened by a contradiction that, he says, was probably a result of having lived through the Depression: his business was growing much faster than anticipated, yet his personal credo did not allow him to turn down new clients.

The holiday was good for Samuel W. He returned to work tan, robust, and refreshed — noticeably content. Mounds of paper had piled up on his desk in his absence; even the sight of them did not alter his upbeat mood.

Unfortunately, his expansiveness was short-lived. Not ten minutes after Samuel W. entered his office a mounting discomfort overtook him. Suddenly his chest was plastered with a pressure heavy as granite that skitted, fanlike and with deliberate, uncompromising motions, across his left side and arms.

His hands and skin became clammy and pale. Dizziness and nausea traveled through him in waves. Sweat poured down his face in large drops. Less than a half-hour later, Samuel W. was at a nearby medical center.

"I was conscious through the whole episode," recalls Samuel W. "I knew damn well I had a heart attack."

What frustrated Samuel W. most about his heart attack was that it drew a line of demarcation separating him from the rest of the world. In that one moment between feeling fresh and alive and feeling desperately ill — in the crucial instant when the bloom of his vacation dissipated into a gray pallor — Samuel W. crossed the boundary dividing those with well bodies and those with bodies in revolt. Samuel W. had become a patient — to his mind, a new category of person — beset by clinical questions and confusing medical nonanswers.

And for the next four years Samuel W. was not spared any confusion about his condition. To begin with, he couldn't get a satisfactory response to the question of why he had suffered his heart attack in the first place. For nearly a decade he had almost obsessively followed the dictates of preventive coronary care; he didn't smoke, drink, eat foods high in LDL cholesterol and triglycerides, or weigh more than the actuarial charts recommend. Still, his cardiac episode that day was massive. A bloodline that feeds the muscle on the front walls of his heart was blocked. In clinical terms, he suffered a myocardial infarct. As a result, Samuel W.'s cardiac ejection fraction, which measures how well the heart is pumping blood, was a mere 20 percent (a normal ejection fraction is 55 percent or higher).

But as bad and incomprehensible as his heart attack was, what followed was numbing. Because of Samuel W.'s age and the advanced disease discovered in his heart, his cardiologists ruled out cardiac bypass surgery, feeling that it would be a life-threatening gamble with few potential rewards. Rather, the physicians prescribed a heart-stabilizing drug to at least thwart Samuel W.'s uncomfortable, but mild, erratic heartbeats — a symptom that emerged as a by-product of his cardiac arrest — while he lived out what they expected to be his last years.

The drug never got a chance to work. Within weeks, Samuel W. had a marked reaction to it in the form of a severe rash that covered his body, and he was taken off the medication. No new medication was prescribed. But without any drugs to stabilize his heart rhythm, for the next two-and-a-half years, Samuel W. suffered a series of discomforting incidents — some were benign, merely dull pains that literally came and went in a matter of seconds; others were breathtaking, dizzying episodes that brought him to the brink of passing out before he just as suddenly recovered.

These attacks were attributed to the unfortunate effects of massive cardiac disease. Sadly, nobody understood that these "nuisance" incidents were of the most insidious sort. Quietly, they were leaving behind an expensive physical debt that would be called in on a hot, humid afternoon in July 1985.

That day, Samuel W.'s children and their families were visiting him and his wife. He was in mid-conversation when, without warning, his heart pitched forward into overdrive and in seconds was pounding at a rate more than three times its normal speed. At one point it was racing at 200 beats per minute.

"I felt as if something otherworldly had taken control of my body and pushed my heart almost to the point of bursting," says Samuel W.

Frightened and sweating profusely, he ran into the bathroom to splash water on his face, to calm the turmoil somehow. But before he stepped out of the bathroom, he blacked out and fell to the floor.

Miraculously, Samuel W. lived through this cardiac electrical storm. And once he was stabilized at the hospital, it took only the briefest of examinations for his physicians to identify what the latest manifestation of Samuel W.'s cardiac disease was all about: his super-rapid pulse, worse than any erratic heartbeat he had suffered before, had been triggered by what became a broadly-based electrical malfunction in his heart known as an arrhythmia.

Unfortunately, knowing the name of his condition and eradicating it were still two entirely different things. Indeed, this was only the beginning for Samuel W. of another series of clinical follies. Over the next nine months, he was alternately put on and then taken off a series of frequently toxic heart drugs. Each of them caused side effects from excruciating aches and pains in his joints that made it almost impossible for him to walk or move to extreme, incapacitating nausea and dizziness.

By February 1986, Samuel W. was a critically ill man; his heart's ejection fraction had slipped to 13 percent, and he suffered from lethargy, fatigue, shortness of breath, low blood pressure, and no appetite. Despite all of the medical attention he had received, he was in far worse condition than four years previously when he suffered his first heart attack. So Samuel W.'s cousin, who lives in Boston, suggested that he be examined by a group of cardiologists at the Massachusetts General Hospital who were using innovative cardiac treatment techniques to restore the hearts of those literally at death's door. Although they relied on methods not at all akin to the traditional strategies of cardiologists, the success rate of these new cardiologists was difficult to ignore.

The trip north was perhaps the best advice Samuel W. received in four years. Miraculously, one laboratory test and one carefully targeted open heart operation later — indeed, in only six weeks — Samuel W. was discharged from Massachusetts General a much healthier man. No drugs were prescribed for his heart rhythm, and once again he was able to resume a more normal life — a little fatigued, perhaps, when exerting himself, but not beset anymore by the constant fear that a new cardiac event was imminent and unsurvivable.

"Looking back, I know I dodged a bullet that packs an enormous amount of punch," says Samuel W.

Actually, he escaped the equivalent of a spray of machine gun fire aimed at his heart.

After Samuel W.'s initial heart attack in 1982, the underlying cause of his recurring symptoms was a repeating, ongoing electrical failure in his heart. Like many doctors adept at traditional cardiology, those who treated Samuel W. were able to diagnose this condition, but they were simply unable to understand its physiological basis and thus never treated him efficaciously. Because of their limited knowledge about new developments in the treatment of abnormal heart rhythms, Samuel W.'s physicians saw no other clinical alternative but the all too commonly used "poke and hope" technique — translated that means prescribing some medication and waiting for subsequent cardiac events, while hoping that they don't occur.

As one cardiologist put it, "That's one of the things that are most distressing about this case. He received standard accepted treatments — and you see what he went through — still his condition deteriorated abysmally."

Samuel W.'s case is not at all atypical. Arrhythmias — the failing and disjointed heart rhythms that plagued and threatened to kill him — are the most pernicious, common, and deadly of all heart conditions. Sadly, it is one of the extreme ironies of modern medicine that arrhythmias are also the heart disease that most cardiologists know the least about.

Consider these facts about arrhythmias:

- They are responsible for over 400,000 sudden deaths each year in this country alone, more than two-thirds of all deaths linked to heart disease; put another way, in the time that it took you to read the previous two paragraphs another person succumbed to arrhythmias.
- Arrhythmias kill more men in the western world than any other disease.
- Annually, only about 100,000 American victims of arrhythmias are resuscitated quickly enough to be around to tell of the ordeal.
- A mere 3,000 arrhythmia patients in the United States each year are fortunate enough to be treated at one of the few medical centers capable of diagnosing and attacking the specific cardiac electrical malfunction from which they suffer.

"We're told so much about the AIDS epidemic that it surprises a lot of people when they hear of the deadly impact of arrhythmias," says Dr. Michel Mirowski, director of the Coronary Care Unit at Sinai Hospital in Baltimore and a professor of medicine at Johns Hopkins University. "But to put it in perspective, we're losing more people in one week from malignant arrhythmias than we've lost from AIDS since the beginning of the epidemic five or six years ago. But nobody is really worried about sudden death from arrhythmias, because the victims die quietly in a rather extreme way; and they don't form pressure groups. It's incomprehensible that the Surgeon General can mention AIDS so often as the most important public health problem and completely ignore arrhythmias."

One of the most devastating types of arrhythmia is known as ventricular tachycardia, a condition in which the heart beats far too fast and does not have enough time to fill its chambers with incoming blood before pumping. The heart ceases to deliver blood to the lungs or throughout the body effectively, and the result is vastly diminished blood pressure or a loss of consciousness and, in some instances, death.

Numerous Holter and electrocardiograph recordings of patients suffering arrhythmias have shown that ventricular tachycardia may be followed by a second electrical disturbance known as ventricular fibrillation. Ventricular fibrillation is a chaotic rhythm in which the pumping chambers of the heart, the ventricles, cease to pump blood altogether. The result, unless treated within seconds, is fatal.

The most common cause of these life-threatening ventricular arrhythmias is any form of damage to the heart muscle, such as ischemia — a dangerous reduction in the blood supply to the heart — or atherosclerosis — a narrowing or blockage of coronary arteries; a cardiac scar, which occurs after a heart attack and after a long interruption of blood flow; and hypertrophy or enlargement of cardiac cells, which is frequently caused by such conditions as severe high blood pressure. In each of these cases, when the heart muscle is compromised, its electrical system is disturbed in the process.

Ventricular tachycardia and fibrillation are deadly time bombs set randomly and silently. In those of us wired to explode they are often undetectable. These arrhythmias are isolated electrical catastrophes that, in those prone to electrical malfunctions of the heart, may occur once a month, once a year, or never in the most fortunate. Moreover, some arrhythmias operate so quietly until they attack with a full frontal assault that, for many, death — sudden and often untimely — caused by an arrhythmia is the first and only manifestation of a heart problem that they will ever have.

The prevalence of life-threatening ventricular arrhythmias, despite resistance, is altering traditional cardiological thought. Although it is difficult to swallow for many in the clinical community, what is being learned about arrhythmias is changing the very notion of what the heart is and how it works: to wit, the heart, it turns out, is *not* merely muscles and blood; rather it *is* a hot-wired organ, dependent on steady and unfailing electrical impulses to perform as an efficient pump.

As Dr. Hasan Garan, codirector of the Cardiac Arrhythmia Service at Massachusetts General, defines the new view of the heart: "The heart is a hotbed of electrical activity, the focal point of electrical impulses arising within its own special pacemaker cells and influenced powerfully by impulses sent from the brain via the nervous system. Once signals arise within the heart, they spread out, ordering the heart's various muscular components to contract or relax in proper sequence. Any disruption of this electrical symphony can have dire, even fatal, results."

The traditional method of treating life-threatening arrhythmias is to prescribe large doses of randomly selected and potentially toxic drugs, as was done for four years in Samuel W.'s case. This technique, time and time again, has failed miserably. Studies have shown that up to 40 percent of arrhythmia patients treated with random, non–carefully guided pharmacologic protocols — that is, the typical way in which drugs are prescribed willy-nilly without diligent laboratory analysis — will have another life-threatening cardiac electrical malfunction within one year, and many will die of it. In fact, approximately one-third of all patients who are resuscitated after out-of-hospital cardiac arrest are found to have been taking anti-arrhythmic drugs at the time of their attack.

But it's not only that incorrectly selected drugs fail to stem arrhythmias. Ironically, they sometimes actually increase the chance of tachycardia and fibrillation.

In short, the drugs are triple-edged swords that can prevent arrhythmias, provoke and exacerbate them, or cause severe toxic side effects, depending on the patient being treated.

"If we have learned one thing in the last ten years," says Dr. Jeremy Ruskin, director of the Cardiac Arrhythmia Service at Massachusetts General and one of the physicians credited with saving Samuel W.'s life, "it is that we cannot reach up on the shelf, pull down a bottle, hand it to a patient with tachycardia and say, 'Here take this and go home. It will work for you,' in the way that we can with penicillin or erythromycin for a streptococcal infection of the throat. Drug therapy for most arrhythmias must be carefully and individually tailored to meet the needs of each patient."

The story of arrhythmias is particularly poignant because not only are they quietly devastating — attacking apparently healthy people like Samuel W. with a blow that can kill in seconds — but often they are self-inflicted. More and more, it appears, our habits and emotions are deadlier than our diseases.

For instance, there has been a frightening upturn recently in the number of sudden cardiac deaths due to arrhythmia among young people and those who ply the upwardly mobile fast track, because of the increasing use of so-called recreational drugs like cocaine and, to a lesser extent, marijuana. The saddest symbol of this group is Len Bias, the man who had, some said, the softest hands in basketball, who for a brief period lived the dream of every playground roundballer by becoming first a University of Maryland All-American and then a Boston Celtic for a day. Ironically, too much success, it is said, was the reason that Bias for all intents and purposes killed himself; he succumbed to a cocaine-induced arrhythmia one early morning in a Baltimore dormitory room.

In addition, common anxiety and stress often contribute to

the sudden onset of arrhythmias in the same way that recreational drugs do. The heart is controlled by nerves. The brain oversees and paces cardiac function, particularly its electrical function; numerous clear signals are delivered to the heart from the sympathetic and parasympathetic nervous systems, two offshoots of the autonomic nervous network, which controls involuntary actions. Any change in brain activity — induced by, for instance, emotional disturbance or depression — affects the quality and nature of nerve traffic that goes to the heart.

Take the case of Charles S., a minister in a rural Tennessee community. Up until recently Charles S. was a withdrawn man. Most of his feelings and personal longings were kept to himself. In many ways, he was the paradigm of the altruistic-to-a-fault, stoic country preacher, a nearly vanished image in this age of Jim Bakker and Jimmy Swaggart. Unbeknown to even his closest friends, he had a very difficult relationship with his wife of thirty years; bickering and anger marked their time together. One day three years ago, Charles S. finally exploded and threw a chair across the room at his wife. Within about an hour, his heart went into ventricular fibrillation so severe that he "dropped dead." Fortunately, he was resuscitated by a nearby physician.

"I was so overwhelmed with guilt," says Charles S. "Here I was a minister preaching peace and nonviolence and the next thing I know I'm trying to kill my wife."

Charles S. is in therapy now. He and his wife have worked through many of their problems and today enjoy a far more open and relaxed relationship. Charles S. has had no recurrence of arrhythmias since that day in 1984.

In many ways the increasing frequency of arrhythmia-victim success stories has been achieved against substantial odds. The new cardiologists taking on our most persistent killer are bucking a health care system and professional attitudes that — in some cases, knowingly, in others, unknowingly — have traditionally resisted change.

To begin with, the medical community has only in recent years come to terms with the devastation caused by arrhythmias. Though sudden death is not a newly discovered phenomenon — its existence has been recognized for centuries — this electrical catastrophe and the damage left in its wake have been accepted by most physicians as an inevitable fact of life about which nothing can be done.

Moreover, slow dissemination of new knowledge about arrhythmias and traditional conservatism in the medical community have influenced the debates over whether anti-arrhythmia treatments and devices are worthy of third-party coverage. Because a majority of all health care costs are now paid by Medicare and other insurance companies, a treatment must be reimbursable to be used frequently and accepted in the medical marketplace. But decisions over which arms of medicine deserve such largesse are generally made by "peer review," advice and consent round tables usually led by veteran physicians. And because, as a whole, the new cardiologists have been viewed as a maverick group by their peers, they have had to battle for scant dollars to keep their fledgling clinical activities afloat.

In the streets and out of the halls of clinical decision making, this new area of cardiology has fared little better. The education of emergency medical teams — the keepers of the front gate in the battle against arrhythmias — about the heart's electrical system and the means to revive patients suffering unexpected cardiac arrest at home or at work has been shamefully slow. Despite a significant recent upturn in federal funding for medical crisis supplies and staffs, fewer than one-third of the rescue squads in the United States are equipped with the knowledge and the tools to save the lives of local residents who collapse suddenly, stricken by arrhythmias.

This situation is particularly distressing because the key to salvaging arrhythmia patients is making certain that they are brought into the hospital alive. Doing this requires extremely timely and appropriate therapy, since a cardiac arrhythmia may be deadly if it is not reversed within minutes. Thus, the fact that most emergency medical units are unable to treat arrhythmias where they occur, before hospital personnel can get involved, ensures that in some districts as many as 90 percent of those who suffer massive electrical heart disturbances at their homes or in the streets will not survive long enough to be cared for by a physician.

Still, despite the bleakness and the obstacles, there is an upside to the story of life-threatening arrhythmias, an upside that is rapidly becoming one of the most significant breakthroughs against disease of this medical era. It was starkly demonstrated in the case of Samuel W., who arrived at Massachusetts General little more than a breath away from death and left with his life renewed.

Propelling this optimism in the fight against the most lethal manifestation of heart disease is a new generation of cardiologists, attacking arrhythmias with nontraditional, inspired solutions. By literally reinducing life-threatening cardiac arrests in those with severe heart disease, these cardiologists are with unwavering determination identifying the code for protecting these patients' hearts against electrical catastrophe.

And as unorthodox as their clinical approach is, the positive statistical results achieved by the new cardiologists are just as unprecedented and equally dramatic: only 10 percent of the critically ill patients they treat have another life-threatening arrhythmia within two years; under the traditional approach, close to 40 percent would have another arrhythmic episode within only one year and many would die of it.

The arrhythmia cardiologists are hybrid scientists, physicians, and engineers, descendants of a long line of researchers in electrophysiology, an esoteric medical science that seeks to understand and use for curative purposes the electrical properties of the human body.

Clinical cardiac electrophysiology has taken root at a number of major medical centers. One of the leading groups in this new effort is at Massachusetts General Hospital. There, Jeremy Ruskin, the physician who led the procedure that saved Samuel W.'s life, keeps a schedule suited only to those attempting to move medical thought squarely and firmly away from its most conservative ideas. Month after month, Ruskin puts in sixty or more hours per week in the wards and laboratory and then takes his act on the road to medical conferences, health care policy seminars, and scientific powwows, pitching the gospel that deadly electrical anomalies of the heart can now be traced, snipped, and rewired; they need not be ignored anymore, nor allowed to have their way with the patient. Ruskin's efforts are paralleled by counterparts at other major arrhythmia centers around the country.

The message of these clinical researchers has not gone unnoticed by the mainstream of cardiologists. Heard more and more are comments like those made by Dr. Enriqué Carter, who sits at the crossroads of conservatism and innovation as the director of the Office of Health Technology Assessment, a branch of the federal Health and Human Services Department: "There are very few people who have the compulsion and the discipline that is required to pursue these new approaches to arrhythmia therapy. It takes nerves of steel to put a critically ill patient into a life-threatening arrhythmia and then rescue him from it. And to use the information gained to figure out how to save his life."

Moreover, spurred by the success of early pilot studies, a number of emergency medical specialists are developing unique prehospital crisis techniques for thwarting arrhythmias and resuscitating patients collapsed from sudden cardiac arrest. Using the latest in emergency medicine techniques, rescue squads in such far-flung places as Seattle, Washington, and Charlottesville, Virginia, are setting a remarkable course by delivering as many as half of the cardiac arrest victims in their districts to the hospital alive, with definitive, invaluable data about their arrhythmia episodes.

Advances in cardiac electrophysiology are occurring so frequently now that researchers are building upon each other's breakthroughs, constructing a ziggurat of medical achievements that none would have thought possible just a decade ago.

As an example, clinical and laboratory investigators have produced computer-created, three-dimensional depictions of the stages and breakdowns in normal performance as a healthy heart deteriorates into an arrhythmic mass of uncadenced muscle.

And on an even more vital plateau that has immediate import for patients with arrhythmias, practical researcher and inventor Dr. Michel Mirowski of Baltimore's Sinai Hospital has created a device called an automatic implantable cardioverter defibrillator (AICD), which has, since it was approved for general use by the U.S. Food and Drug Administration in December 1985, exceeded all expectations. A three-inch wide piece of titanium that is embedded under a patient's skin near the abdomen and plugged into the heart with electrodes, the AICD continuously monitors the electrical activity of the ventricles. When the internal rhythm becomes dangerously fast, without prompting the device delivers a countershock that normalizes the pulse beat. The one-year arrhythmia mortality rate of patients with arrhythmias who have had cardioverter defibrillators installed is a meager 2 percent.

Heart Rhythms is a story of patients and individual heartbeats and of disciplined physicians and researchers emerging as disease slayers. Enlivening the story are patients ranging from those with the riskiest of life-styles to those living God-fearing lives in the hamlets; the intricacies of chance and discovery as they form the foundation of the latest high and low technologies to fight our most lethal disease; and the vastly complicated battles over cost, turf, and ideas that currently suffuse medicine. But beyond all of that, *Heart Rhythms* is, at its core, a book of practical new medical information that could save your life or the lives of those you love.

·2·

The Heart Electric

F ORGET everything you learned in school about the heart. Though no biology or anatomy teacher ever even hinted at it, the vaunted pump is merely a slave to electricity.

Electrical signals from two sets of antagonistic nerves regulate the pumping action of the heart (Figure 1). The sympathetic nerves, which branch out from a series of lateral cells in the spinal cord, are the source of stimulation when a faster and stronger pulse beat is required. For instance, if an athlete is taxing the body with a strenuous feat, these nerves send a message to the heart that its contracting force must be increased. A larger volume of blood is relayed to the body to pay the oxygen debt incurred during the activity.

On the other hand, the vagus nerve, which emerges from the cardiac center in the medulla oblongata, the lower portion of the brainstem, is called upon at those times when slower and less powerful heartbeats are to be produced.

As in all nervous activity, electrochemical transmitters, in this case acetylcholine and norepinephrine, carry the messages of the vagus and sympathetic neurons.

The Nervous System of the Heart

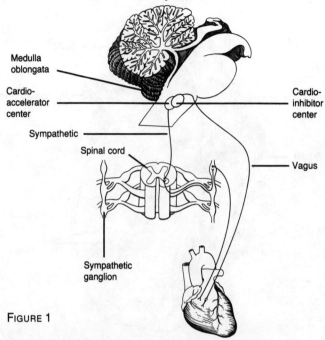

Medulla oblongata

Cardio-accelerator center

Cardio-inhibitor center

Sympathetic

Spinal cord

Vagus

Sympathetic ganglion

FIGURE 1

Electrical impulses originate within the heart at the sinoatrial node, known as the pacemaker of the heart because it is here that the normal heartbeat begins (Figure 2). The sinoatrial node is located at the top of the right atrium, where blood returning from the body also initiates its cardiac journey.

From the sinoatrial node, impulses are transmitted to the heart's upper, priming chambers, the right and left atria, and then to the atrioventricular node. The atrioventricular node is at the junction of the atria and the heart's lower, pumping chambers, the ventricles. Importantly, it is the sole electrical connection between the heart's upper and lower chambers.

From here the electrical waves are conducted to the bundle of His and the Purkinje fibers, both weaves of specialized cardiac muscle that snake through the working muscles of the ventricles. His and Purkinje fibers are adapted for very rapid conduction of electrical impulses and can transmit a charge throughout the heart's lower chambers in milliseconds.

Three special properties of the heart's electrical system co-

The Electrical Conduction System of the Heart

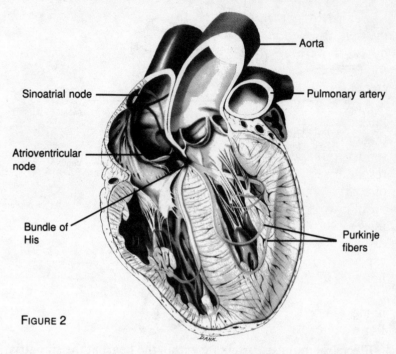

Aorta

Sinoatrial node

Pulmonary artery

Atrioventricular node

Bundle of His

Purkinje fibers

FIGURE 2

ordinate the pumping action of its four chambers and turn this mass of muscle into an efficient pump. First, at the atrioventricular node, a delay is introduced so that electrical signals are transmitted to the ventricles on a jazzlike "back beat," ensuring that the lower chambers do not contract and attempt to discharge blood to the lungs or the body until they have become filled with blood from the atria.

Second, the bundle of His and the Purkinje fibers carrying this pulse through the ventricles communicate an entire network of muscular activity through interwoven points of contact at specialized cells. When a fiber is in the resting state, the electrical potential inside the cell membrane is lower, or more negative, than the one outside the membrane. What stimulates this fiber into contraction is the rapid flow of several ions across the cell's outer membrane, making the cell interior positive for a brief instant. Then, just as rapidly, the positive charge inside the cell dissipates and the fiber is quiescent again. Thus, fueled by the rush of ions across cell membranes, the atria and ventricles contract and rest in a coordinated rhythmic fashion to create the pumping action of the heart.

And third, the electrical stimulation of the bundle of His and Purkinje fibers is extremely long in duration compared with that of the body's skeletal muscles. Because of this, the heart's refractory period, when it will not respond to stimuli, is correspondingly elongated. This creates the exaggerated cadences of contraction and relaxation unique to the heart.

An arrhythmia occurs when the elegant cell-to-cell communication and fiber-to-fiber wiring scheme of the heart are disturbed. Isolated electrical impulses start suddenly and unexpectedly in the atria or ventricles, rather than through the normal activation pathway that begins in the sinoatrial node.

Cardiac arrhythmias are extremely common, and most are not at all life threatening or indicative of any physical problems. For instance, we've all experienced the sensation of the heart skipping a beat. Physiologically, this occurs because a ventricle is stimulated out of synch by an errant impulse inside the chamber. When the normal electrical charge arrives from the atrium, the ventricle is still recovering from its premature impulse and cannot respond effectively. Thus, the ventricle will ignore the atrium's electrical transmission this time and await another activation sequence before pumping blood into the lungs or body. It feels like a missed beat, a rough cadence waiting to be smoothed. Usually an isolated incident that occurs infrequently, this type of arrhythmia is of little concern.

Life-threatening arrhythmias, on the other hand, are continuous, unflagging skipped beats strung together to cause ventricular tachycardia or fibrillation. They occur when the ventricles are repeatedly stimulated at a rate of between 140 and 300 electrical impulses — heartbeats — per minute. This might occur because scar tissue due to cardiac disease — known or unknown — has begun to interfere with the heart's normal electrical activation pattern and, in effect, usurps the intrinsic design and sets up its own impulse pathways. Or it can be the result of a transient reduction in blood flow to the ventricles, known as ischemia. But, whatever the cause, rapid heartbeats and jacked up contractions in the ventricles lead to vastly diminished cardiac output, because not enough blood has been received by the pumping chamber before it attempts to transfer it to the body. Circulatory collapse, loss of consciousness, and, frequently, death follow.

This type of tachycardia often degenerates into ventricular fibrillation, entirely asynchronous and chaotic electrical activity. Ventricular fibrillation is extremely life threatening; more than two-thirds of all deaths from arrhythmia are caused by it.

The basic understanding that physicians have today about these ventricular arrhythmias, their genesis in an individual, and their modus operandi, has chiefly emerged during the past decade. But it is the culmination of two hundred years of research, gathered in small and large pieces, about the electrical properties of the human body in general and the heart in particular. The first clues were uncovered in the eighteenth century.

By the middle of that century, the age of electricity was in full bloom. In 1752, Benjamin Franklin performed his famous kite experiment in Philadelphia; a professor in St. Petersburg, Russia, was electrocuted independently attempting the same feat with a poorly insulated lightning rod; and numerous sideshows and carnivals offered patrons a chance for them and their neighbors to experience a group shock by sharing a line of charged wire.

The worldwide preoccupation with things electrical inspired more than just general interest. It spawned a new science, electrophysiology, founded by a cadre of physicians intrigued enough to wonder whether electricity played a role in anatomical processes. Taking note of electricity's significant effect on the body, these doctors pondered the obvious: are electrical currents inside our bodies the unknown force that powers muscular motion? Perhaps, they mused, electricity, which has such an immediate and unmistakable impact on the human body, holds the secret of movement.

Before long, these physicians had at least a partial answer to their ruminations. In 1770, in the laboratory of an Italian doctor, Louis Galvani, it was discovered that electricity was indeed capable of stimulating contraction of the muscles. It began quite by chance, when Galvani prepared to dissect a frog to study its anatomy and placed it on a table which held a crude friction machine that produced electrical currents.

"One of my assistants accidentally lightly applied the point of a scalpel to the frog's inner crural nerves," wrote Galvani. "Suddenly, all of the muscles of the limbs were seen so to contract that they appeared to have fallen into violent tonic convulsions. Meantime, another assistant . . . thought he observed that this occurred when a spark was discharged from the conductor of the electrical machine."

Upon further examination, Galvani found that his assistant had jarred the friction machine only slightly as he prepared to touch the frog. A low-level current was transmitted to the scalpel in his hand and then to the amphibian's nerve. Galvani repeated this experiment on the frog and again the frog convulsed.

For its time, this was a remarkable discovery. By focusing electricity on an animal's nerve, Galvani had actually made its body move. His experiment caused electricity to be regarded with increased respect and awe. Some saw it as a physical force emanating like lightning bolts directly from the hands of God. What's more, many electrophysiologists were satisfied that their suspicions were not unfounded: Galvani's experiment seemed to corroborate their notion that electricity is, indeed, the orchestrator of movement on earth.

Word of Galvani's experience with the twitching frog spread quickly throughout the electrophysiological and medical communities. An era began in which electricity was seen as one of the essences of life and even as a cure-all. Physicians and quacks alike administered shock treatments to patients for ailments ranging from the most common to the most insidious. Doctors reported some clinical success with electrotherapy, especially in cases of "sluggish respiration and sluggish circulation," as one British doctor noted.

Initially, electricity was not used for resuscitation but only as a tonic or a stimulant. However, it would not be long before electricity was put to work to revive collapsed bodies, as Humane Societies sprang up all over Europe and the United States dedicated "to the resuscitation [with electricity] of persons apparently dead." So, in 1774, when a London boy fell out a window and stopped breathing, a Mr. Squires of Soho applied an electrical shock to the five-year-old's chest. Remarkably, the boy was successfully revived.

The tabloids and the responsible press had a field day with this incident: God's mysterious physical force had actually saved a lost soul — and a child's at that. Though it was, of course, not understood then, the explanation for what happened is one of the tenets of clinical arrhythmia cardiology today. The electrical shock normalized or, in current medical terminology, defibrillated the boy's cardiac fibrillation, his arrhythmia.

Following the reports of this case, electrophysiologists developed a crude defibrillating device for resuscitating persons. It consisted only of two electrodes that conducted electricity stored in a Leyden jar, an early version of the battery. With this unit, numerous attempts followed to resuscitate those who died from any cause, not just cardiac shock, such as the boy suffered, or heart attacks. Some victims were revived; many, much to the chagrin of electrophysiologists and sideshow barkers alike, never budged.

Dabbling in defibrillation reached its apex — and its nadir — in 1820, when the portable reanimation or resuscitation chair was designed. To use this macabre device, a physician strapped a collapsed patient into the chair and plugged his ears with cotton. Then a mouthpiece was secured between the patient's teeth through which one electrode was passed and attached to the stomach and another to the larynx. A third electrode was placed on the outside of the patient's body, usually on the thorax. Finally, an electrical charge was delivered that was so severe that the patient's body was nearly catapulted out of the contraption.

Needless to say, this precursor to the electric chair did little to save lives. The damage from the electrodes hastily shoved into the patient's body and from the penetrating electrical shock — not to mention the time it took to set the patient up in the chair — mitigated against resuscitation. With the failures of the resuscitation chair, the period's love affair with defibrillation dissipated rather quickly.

Still, what came out of the early resuscitation efforts with electricity was empirical evidence that the body's muscles responded to electrical impulses. Under certain conditions, it was clear that electrical currents excited "dead" persons back to life. From this discovery, suspicions persisted that because the heart is the pump of life, it was probably the organ that responded to electroshock in those instances in which resuscitation was successful. But without X rays, fluoroscopes, and open heart experimentation this was extremely difficult to prove.

In 1855, though, two Danish physicians offered the initial proof of the electrophysiological properties of the heart by demonstrating that it contained an electrical current. They removed a nerve-muscle combination from a frog's leg and placed the end of the neuron on the surface of a beating heart. With every systole, or contraction, of the ventricle the muscle jerked. Moreover, a second feeble twitch was observed at the beginning of every diastole, or ventricular, refractory period. Because it was already known from Galvani's work that electrical impulses were the impetus for the movement of muscles, the Danes concluded correctly that in their experiment it must be electrical impulses from the heart that caused the twitching of the frog muscle. For the first time, the existence of a pure cardiac electrical current had been proved by segregating and identifying it.

The next logical step would have been to describe cardiac electrical properties more distinctly, by detailing intensity variations of different parts of the heart during separate stages of the pulse beat, the way an electrocardiogram (in medical short-hand, an EKG) does. But unfortunately, the tools available at that time were simply too crude to permit this.

As one physician noted in frustration, "The phenomena we can observe and not merely hypothesize about are limited by the instruments we employ rather than by the organs we explore." Still, the Danish experiment, by simply proving that the heart has a powerful electrical charge, is credited as the first primitive step toward the development of an electrocardiograph that could analyze the heart from its electrical output and ultimately denote the presence and seriousness of arrhythmias.

The development of the electrocardiograph would have to wait only twenty years. By 1876, the invention of a new device known as the capillary electrometer, which contained mercury and sulfuric acid and measured the rise and fall of electrical pressure, enabled the French-born English physician Augustus Waller to design a primitive electrocardiograph to record the electrical activity of the beating heart.

Waller's classic demonstration of his electrocardiograph took place in his laboratory at London's St. Mary's Hospital in May. Before a group of distinguished physiologists, Waller tethered a patient to a six-foot-tall metal box by placing electrodes on his chest and back. Then, using the capillary electrometer in the massive electrocardiograph, he demonstrated how the heart's electrical output rose and fell throughout the pulse beat. This was a significant breakthrough in that, for the first time, an electrical analysis of the heart was obtained. However, Waller's electrocardiograph was of little clinical value, as it became clear almost immediately that the capillary electrometer was unable to discern most subtle cardiac electrical activity; its measuring electrodes were stymied by having to read the true heart beat through the diffuse layers of skin and muscle. Thus, Waller's results were rife with errors and misreadings.

However, one of the physiologists at Waller's laboratory that day, the German William Einthoven, recognized the potential importance of the electrocardiograph as a diagnostic and investigative tool. He devoted the next twenty years of his life to upgrading Waller's device. And by the end of the century Einthoven had designed an electrocardiograph that was much more sophisticated than Waller's. Not only was it extremely accurate, it was also portable, at least in the sense that it could be stored in a large clinic away from the hospital rooms and through wires read the patient's heart rhythms even while the patient lay in bed on the ward.

The key to the success of Einthoven's electrocardiograph was that the electrodes were improved sufficiently so that their measuring antennae cut through the resistance offered by the body's skin and muscles. Upon examining the distinct accuracy of this electrocardiograph's tracings, Waller had to admit grudgingly: "Einthoven's machine is to mine as a high-powered microscope is to a low-powered microscope. It has opened a new chapter in the clinical study of heart disease, and played a part in medical literature that should far exceed the fact that it was created by electrophysiology."

This statement is a reflection of the fact that, at the time, electrophysiologists were no darlings of mainstream clinicians. A rift had grown separating those physicians preferring traditional — often passive — cardiac treatments and diagnostic methods and those who felt that the way to understand the nature of the heart's physiology and diseases was to uncover its electrical properties.

Still, as Waller had hoped, Einthoven's electrocardiograph achieved acclaim. Physicians applauded his achievement while they continued to ignore and downplay the importance of most other discoveries of the early electrophysiologists. In 1924, two years after Waller's death in relative obscurity, Einthoven was awarded the Nobel prize in physiology and medicine "for the discovery of the mechanism of the electrocardiogram."

To many in the medical community, the electrocardiograph stands out as the one lasting achievement of the electrophysiologists in the late 1800s, but that could not be farther from the truth. Indeed, to understand how far the electrophysiologists had progressed in uncovering the characteristics of cardiac electrical disease, even before the advent of sophisticated equipment like Einthoven's, consider that the term *arrhythmia* was coined as early as 1875 by the physiologist Rudolf Heidenhain; it was used as a catchall, one-word description for every disturbance of cardiac rhythm. Relying on nothing more than simple tactile examination of pulse beats, electrophysiologists noted that certain compounds like chloroform — used then as an anesthetic during the extraction of teeth — produced a rapid heart rate, which, in turn, sometimes led to shock and even death.

Soon after Heidenhain invented the name, an arrhythmia was "seen" for the first time, when the physician John A. MacWilliam of the University of Aberdeen identified the electrical signatures of arrhythmias. MacWilliam came upon the picture of an arrhythmia during experiments he conducted in response to the growing concern over electrocution, which was becoming more and more prevalent with the development of industrial high-current electrical motors. Using Waller's less-than-perfect electrocardiograph, MacWilliam shocked to death a group of animals and then printed out a series of EKGs covering their last breaths. Depicted were the tall, bunched lines of ventricular fibrillation — then known as delirium cordis, madness of the heart — as the final spasms of their lives.

Translating freely from his animal studies, MacWilliam added that when such an arrhythmia occurs in people, either during electrocution or naturally, the result is sudden cardiac arrest. During these deaths, he said, the heart does not simply stop, but enters into violent and disorganized activity.

By this point, electrophysiologists were so enamored with what they were learning about arrhythmias that implanting electrodes in the hearts of animals and shocking them to death was commonplace and frequent. Not a detail of the frenzied electrocuted heart was left unexamined. This was made especially clear by the writings of Drs. Willis Tacker, Jr., and Leslie Geddes of Purdue University, who described in graphic prose the tactile sensations of an arrhythmic, dying heart.

When a fibrillating heart is held in the hand, it feels like a wad of writhing worms. In many cases, the rate of this random process is so rapid that the heart surface seems to shimmer. In other instances, multiple waves of contraction and relaxation are clearly visible.

Still, despite the achievements of the electrophysiologists in the late 1800s, using crude or no medical instrumentation, it wasn't until the arrival of Einthoven's electrocardiograph that these physicians unearthed one of the most peculiar and important properties of arrhythmia: there is a short window of opportunity during which an arrhythmia can be reversed by a separate, carefully timed electrical shock, an interval when, ironically, the current that kills could, in proper doses, be the current that saves.

In the 1920s two European physicians, J. L. Prevost and F. Battelli, grew curious about whether this revival period existed, when they examined the records of the resuscitation efforts in the late 1700s. Some people, like the young British boy who had fallen out the window and was revived by a shock from an electrode, had actually been brought back to life. What was the physiological mechanism that permitted this? they wondered.

So Prevost and Battelli painstakingly attached an electrocardiograph's electrodes to frog after frog, electrocuted the animals, and then jolted them with a second dose of electricity just as the EKG showed they were having the ventricular fibrillation that could kill them. It took many attempts, but in time the researchers were able to identify the exact moment when the arrhythmia could be normalized by the electrical shock. And over a period of years more and more test frogs lived through these laboratory brushes with electrocution.

From MacWilliam's earlier work with electrocution, electrophysiologists had proof that ventricular fibrillation existed and that it was deadly, but now they had proof of a method for counteracting it. Prevost's and Battelli's experiments were seminal in arrhythmia research — and continue to play a leading role in the diagnosis and treatment of the condition. As a direct result of their clinical research, people collapsing on street corners today may be fortunate enough to arrive at the hospital alive and with a normal heart rhythm. These two physicians proved that arrhythmias — caused by electricity at its most damaging — can be reversed by electricity at its most curative.

Ventricular fibrillation is but one of the many possible arrhythmias, and with the aid of Einthoven's electrocardiograph, Sir Thomas Lewis, from 1915–1925, amassed the official EKG gallery of all electrical fluctuations of the heart. Through observation upon observation and careful filtering of the data, every conceivable type of arrhythmia — from those of atrial origin to those originating in the atrioventricular node and in the ventricles themselves — was analyzed and described by its electrical waves.

For instance, Lewis made the initial electrocardiographic description of ventricular tachycardia on a patient with shortness of breath, chest pains, and dropsy, a condition in which an excessive amount of fluid lies fallow in the tissues. Lewis described this particular tachycardia in explicit detail, portraying it as a ventricular anomaly with three to eleven successive rapid and abnormal heart beats produced by aberrant cardiac electrical activation cycles. This EKG was a critical advance. While it was already understood that arrhythmias were the result of such accidents as electrocution and while it was assumed that they were also a subset of cardiac disease, Lewis had finally produced proof in the form of an EKG that a sick heart was frequently an arrhythmic heart.

By this point the electrophysiologists were clearly on to something major. There finally was growing evidence that ventricular arrhythmias killed and killed often, that they were a crippling manifestation of heart disease, and that they could be reverted by a carefully planted jolt of electricity. But few electrophysiologists were game enough to try their new-found notions out on people. Unlike the designers of the reanimation chair in the early 1800s, these scientists were facing a far too inhospitable medical climate to risk severe rebuke by attempting to right an arrhythmia through electrotherapy. The schism between traditional doctors and electrophysiologists had widened rapidly after the traditional medical community took the EKG for its own diagnostic purposes, while ignoring the other precepts and ideas of the discipline from which it emerged. Thus, it would take another twenty years of intense laboratory experimentation before an electrophysiologist corrected the arrhythmia of a human patient.

The 1920s through the 1940s were watershed years for arrhythmia research, because during this time its theater changed from Europe to the United States. Although up to this point much of the arrhythmology advances had been made in England, Germany, France, and Italy, the more frequent scientific and cultural exchanges of this period between Europe and America, a by-product of World War I, changed all that. Many of the American physicians and electrophysiologists who went to Europe because of the war sought out legends like Thomas Lewis, became swept up by the elegance of their findings and the years of experience summed up in their anecdotes, and brought this information back to the United States.

After the completion of his last book of arrhythmias, in 1924, Sir Thomas Lewis tired of the subject and turned his attention away from the heart. According to his confidants, Lewis believed that the electrocardiogram had yielded all it could about arrhythmias by this point and that he would do well to put his energies into other medical pursuits. Never again would this clinical scientist be so ambitious or successful.

By the 1930s, the body of information that the electrophysiologists had amassed about arrhythmias was substantial. And the next twenty years are best known for two conceptual discoveries that — like the work of Prevost and Battelli — would still influence the clinical community decades later and become central parts of the clinical foundation that today's cardiologists rely on to assess and treat arrhythmias.

The first has to do with arrhythmia drug therapies. It came

to light in 1930, when the American physiologist William Strauss took the mountains of electrocardiographic information available about ventricular arrhythmias and created a statistical fact sheet describing typical arrhythmia sufferers.

He analyzed sixty-four patients with ventricular tachycardia. Sixty percent were males between 50 and 60 years old; 83 percent showed scarred cardiac muscle and 66 percent suffered from a severely diminished output of blood from the heart. Interestingly, while this report was based on very limited data, Strauss's portrait of the severe ventricular arrhythmia patient does not differ in any significant ways from similar analyses conducted today.

But perhaps Strauss's most interesting discovery was that in 50 percent of the cases, digitalis, then a frequently used drug for the treatment of heart disease, was administered right before the onset of tachycardia. This was a disturbing finding, especially since mainstream cardiologists — that is, nonelectrophysiologists — were caring for almost all arrhythmia victims and the cardiologists' normal protocol was to prescribe drugs like digitalis. However, with Strauss's observations and the work of others it became apparent that the use of excessive amounts of digitalis seemed to play a significant role in actually precipitating arrhythmias.

Not long after Strauss's research, a somewhat overly aggressive experiment provided further early proof that drugs commonly used for arrhythmias are, at worst, dangerous and, at best, unpredictable. Dr. James Scott had a patient who suffered episodes of ventricular tachycardia each time he exercised strenuously. So, Scott decided to use this patient as a human laboratory. He administered an anti-arrhythmia drug to him, then asked the patient to jog in place. His goal was to determine which pharmacotherapy, if any, could keep the patient's cardiac rhythms normal during uninhibited exercise.

Scott repeated this investigation numerous times, testing a variety of prescriptions. Digitalis, atropine, and epinephrine all failed to stem the tachycardia. Quinidine, on the other hand, a fairly new drug at that time, both terminated and prevented the patient's arrhythmic episodes.

What Scott's experiment hinted at is something that continues to haunt and confuse arrhythmia specialists today. It is an unexplainable medical anomaly; for some patients there are benign, nontoxic drugs that can shut down their arrhythmic symptoms, but there is no formula to match the correct drug with a given patient. From one patient to the next the response to different anti-arrhythmia drugs is highly varied and unpredictable. A good bookmaker could set odds on whether a chosen pharmacotherapy will save a life or be impotent in the face of a particular patient's recurrent arrhythmia; the outcome is completely in doubt.

Essentially, to the eyes of medical men, whether a drug is efficacious or not is a problem in random statistical analysis, ironically as random as the moment when an incipient arrhythmia attacks. In fact, more than anything else perhaps, it is the terrible unknowns inherent in arrhythmia drug protocols that goad today's arrhythmia cardiologists to find alternate, nonpharmaceutical means to deal with the devastating condition.

Unfortunately, Scott's underlying message about the disparate behavior of arrhythmia drugs was lost on most cardiologists. Instead, relying on the more overt results of Scott's research and other independent analyses, they made quinidine the drug of choice for most ventricular arrhythmias. As could be expected, though, quinidine was no more a panacea than any other arrhythmia drug. And in a short time many cardiologists became concerned about the increasingly frequent examples of quinidine toxicity among their patients, but not concerned enough to stop prescribing it.

As one physician wrote in the *Journal of the American Medical Association:* "The fact that the patient becomes nauseated, dizzy, weak, or develops diarrhea or ringing of the ears should not discourage the physician from persisting with this therapy, when the alternative is likely to be fatal termination."

Before long, any logic in this statement became hollow. Although quinidine continues to be a widely used and effective drug for the treatment of arrhythmias, its use is associated with significant potential for toxicity.

The second conceptual breakthrough of the 1930s occurred on an entirely different front. Some electrophysiologists felt that the EKG did not deliver enough hard information about the exact location of arrhythmias; the EKG instead only identified the presence of tachycardia and fibrillation in a generalized fashion, ascribing it to a broad rather than a specific locale. They thought that to design a treatment method for a patient's arrhythmias, nothing less than the particular site at which they strike the heart had to be pinpointed.

Thus, in the late 1920s Dr. Werner Forssmann set out to devise a method to locate heart arrhythmias. The era of so-called intracardiac recordings — measurements taken from inside the heart as opposed to views obtained from the chest's outer skin — was launched. In his research Forssmann used himself as the lab animal. He inserted a catheter with an electrode into his own femoral artery and snaked it through the blood vessel until it reached the ventricle of his heart. Forssmann listened closely to what the electrode could "hear" and discern from the pulsating ventricle.

Unfortunately, the electrode picked up nothing but random, indeterminate background sounds; audio-filtering technology was simply not advanced enough to ignore "noise" and focus solely on cardiac artifacts. Forssmann was frustrated by the failure of his experiment. He concluded that the idea that internal cardiac signals could be picked up by an invasive exploratory electrode was flawed and would never be implemented.

However, even in his lack of success Forssmann had provided an essential glimmer of the clinical future. Soon after, somewhat noisy, but decipherable, intracardiac currents were for the first time retrieved through catheters by André Cournand and Dickinson Richards, two cardiologists at Columbia-Presbyterian Medical Center in New York City. And finally, in the mid-1950s, properly designed filters that remove much of the localized cardiac "noise" from recordings enabled these researchers and other electrophysiologists to produce intracardiac readings that were clear and precise and even to detect the exact location of arrhythmias. This technology is the bedrock of arrhythmia cardiology.

But of all the chronological landmarks in electrophysiology, 1947 stands out. That year a long-held suspicion of electrophysiologists and arrhythmia researchers was tested in an operating room on a human being, and the outcome was successful.

The conclusion that a fibrillating heart could be normalized or defibrillated by a jolt of electricity had been demonstrated on frogs twenty years earlier by Prevost and Battelli but never on people. Since then, electrophysiologists, hoping to hurry the day when a cardiologist would have the stomach and sheer will to test defibrillation on humans, had been rigging up all kinds of devices to countershock arrhythmias in the operating room. Finally, one of these devices was used during an anxious moment by Dr. Claude Beck, a young cardiac surgeon at Case Western Reserve Hospital in Cleveland.

Among cardiologists, Beck was an outcast. He was seen less as a maverick electrophysiologist and more as a self-absorbed, limelight-seeking, aggressive surgeon who attempted to save lives with far too much abandon. Most cardiologists felt that Beck could not define the boundary between treating a patient with proper clinical strategies and outright tampering with life and death. His Hippocratic oath was said by some to be "all hearts are too good to die." A joke making the rounds of cardiology circles during Beck's life was, "When you faint in Cleveland near Beck's operating room, you'll awaken with a bloody shirt."

But Beck would make medical history on a cold and cloudy day in 1947. His patient was a fourteen-year-old boy who had severe and critical disease of the pericardium, the thin fibrous sac that surrounds the heart. To save the teenager's life, Beck, practicing his own dubious form of cardiology, decided to remove part of the youth's pericardium. At best this procedure would add a short time to the dying boy's life; at worst, it would kill him.

Dr. Gordon Moe recalls Beck's activities in the operating room that day well. Moe is one of the grand old men of arrhythmia research and one of the few still alive to talk about the seminal years in electrophysiology that spanned the 1930s and 1940s. At the time of Beck's operation on the fourteen-year-old boy, Moe was also at Case Western, a graduate student just beginning his medical career under the tutelage of the physiologist Carl Wiggers.

"The only reason why Beck had the defibrillator in his operating room is because Carl Wiggers gave him one not long before," Moe says. "Wiggers told Beck, 'You may not ever have occasion to use this, but here is the instrument we use in the laboratory to restore a normal rhythm during experiments with animals that have arrhythmic hearts. Keep it near you. Some day you'll save a life.' "

Beck was fortunate to have Wigger's defibrillator close at hand that day. Ignoring the repeated advice of electrophysiologists, Beck gave the boy massive doses of digitalis, until he was literally poisoned by the drug. Beck reasoned that his patient needed the drug to maintain his heart's strength during the operation. Unfortunately, though, the contra-indication of the medication — specifically, its tendency to cause arrhythmias when taken by the wrong patient — applied to the boy.

So as soon as Beck started excising the teenager's pericardium, the heart tumbled into ventricular fibrillation and immediately stopped pumping. In panic Beck reached for Wigger's defibrillator, put the electrodes on the boy's heart, and delivered an enormous shock that miraculously rocketed his rhythm back to normal.

It was an ironic operation. A near miss in his operating room — a result of his own mishandling of the case — a flirtation with death, and Beck was suddenly the toast of much of the medical community. Against all odds, Beck had actually brought a patient back from the dead using a defibrillator, proving a theory that had previously been much maligned by the mainstream medical community.

Beck wrote paper after paper about his "achievement" and spoke about the operating room miracle at every conference of physicians that he could attend. His name became synonymous with the best of electrophysiology and the avant-garde of arrhythmia research. Strangely, although it was dubious medicine that led to the use of the defibrillator, what happened in Beck's operating room that day went a long way toward legitimizing much of arrhythmia research.

The irony is only compounded when you consider the primitive, homemade gadget Beck used on his patient for defibrillation. The electrodes were two hammered-out copper spoons wrapped in gauze, each with a wire dipped in concentrated salt solution and plugged into a 60-cycle electrical line receiving power from three one-hundred watt light bulbs.

Still, Beck's antics in the operating room were essential to electrophysiologists; his experiment precipitated at least a slight closing of the breach that separated them from traditional cardiologists, a breach that Gordon Moe remembers most vividly. Most physicians, Moe recalls, had nothing but antipathy for researchers investigating the devastation of arrhythmias.

"When I told people that I decided to learn under Carl Wiggers they told me to my face — and with no embarrassment," says Moe, " 'Why would you go spend a year to work with Carl Wiggers? You're going to be studying arrhythmias — fibrillation and tachycardia — and nothing can be done about them anyway. You'll be wasting your time.' "

Time after time in those years this attitude reared its head. At a meeting of thoracic surgeons, for instance, an ad hoc discussion began about techniques for ventricular defibrillation, but the chairman interrupted the dialogue, saying that "surgeons had no use for such prattle."

"To see the deep schism between electrophysiologists and clinical cardiologists you just have to look at the makeup of the American Heart Association through these years," notes

Moe. "From its inception in the nineteen-twenties until the late nineteen-forties, I don't think there was a single electrophysiologist in the group. Finally, when the basic science council, an advanced research group, was formed by Carl Wiggers, among others, in the late 1940s, the AHA became more than a mainstream clinical cardiologist's club.

"The problem was that the mainstream cardiologists were nothing more than clinicians who essentially practiced medicine according to recipe books. They were useless to so many of their patients. If a patient had a complaint, the physician would look up the diagnosis in the *Merck Index* and prescribe the drug that was recommended for treating it. No recognition was given to the essential underlying physical foundation of the patient's problem."

Moe says that what gratified him most was that while established physicians never sought out his advice and medical students — modeling themselves in a perverse way on the oldest traditions of medicine, even if those traditions lacked modern wisdom — also avoided his counsel, the house staff working in the trenches, on the wards with the patients, often asked him questions about how to treat patients with intractable heart arrhythmias.

"They were faced with reality," Moe notes. "Life and death. Hearts that beat out of cadence and no help in sight. When they looked at these patients they wished they understood physiology a lot better."

The ultimate problem of dealing with arrhythmias, according to Moe, is that they are so devious and resistant to generalizations. Now "an old and diseased man," as he describes himself, Moe says that what he knows after all his years in arrhythmia research is that the new cardiologists who are fighting arrhythmias today are aiming at a swiftly moving target and their success is testimony to sheer persistence in the face of uncommonly poor odds.

"When I left Wiggers's lab, I thought I knew all there was to know about cardiac arrhythmias and about the treatment of cardiac arrhythmias," he says. "I should have stopped there.

But the more research I did the less I could honestly say I knew about the intricate mechanisms of arrhythmias. I have learned, for example, that almost all of the anti-arrhythmic drugs are also capable of causing arrhythmias. So it's a matter of very delicate judgment and clinical stubbornness to treat a disease as powerful as arrhythmias."

· 3 ·

Serendipity at Columbia-Presbyterian

B Y the 1960s, the electrophysiologists had come a long way. They had proved — though few other cardiologists were listening — that arrhythmias are a substantial cardiac problem, often the underlying pathology in heart disease. And in Claude Beck's unlikely operating room, a patient with a "fatal" arrhythmia had been miraculously revived by a therapeutic dose of electricity.

Beck's defibrillation led to numerous other attempts to countershock arrhythmic human hearts in laboratories and operating rooms around the country. Most were successful. Indeed, in 1962, while it could not be called common, it was still not unusual for a patient near cardiac death to have his heart defibrillated with electroshock before drugs and other more traditional protocols were prescribed. Like arrhythmias themselves, which were once considered cardiac nuisances about which nothing could be done and therefore worthy of little clinical research, defibrillation — electrical engineering, not medicine, to many cardiologists — was finally being given its due by mainstream cardiologists.

Cheryl S. was one who survived only because of electro-shock. The sixty-three-year-old Boston housewife was vacuuming early one afternoon when she abruptly suffered a severe crushing chest pain. It subsided and she ignored it. Over the next two weeks she continued to clean her home, cook, shop, and run errands. But she had constant dyspnea, a condition in which breathing becomes more and more difficult. Then, while resting one afternoon, she suddenly collapsed.

When she arrived at nearby Peter Bent Brigham Hospital, her respiration had slowed measurably; her neck veins were engorged and her abdomen distended as she perpetually tried to catch her breath. But it was Cheryl S.'s heart rate that told the true story of her condition: it was streaking along at a consistent 200 beats per minute. She was suffering a classic ventricular tachycardia and suffocating from it. Her heart rate was too rapid to output sufficient amounts of blood to maintain the blood pressure and to feed the cells with enough oxygen.

Initial treatment in the hospital centered on the use of drugs and, as happens so often, it failed. Cheryl S. was given procainamide hydrochloride, then potassium chloride, and finally quinidine. Her heartbeat refused to slow. From time to time it actually sped up. Watching her condition worsen, literally by the second, Brigham electrophysiologists like Dr. Bernard Lown argued that the only way to save Cheryl S.'s life was by reverting her arrhythmia with a countershock. Backed against a wall, confused, and not sure what other treatment to turn to next, her physicians finally assented.

Cheryl S. was anesthetized and jolted with a single 100 watt-second discharge; immediately her heart rate returned to normal. Within several minutes, her pulmonary congestion disappeared entirely. A few minutes later Cheryl S. was awake.

One of the physicians in attendance recalls, "She looked startled, like she was awakened from a bad dream in which she was convinced that she was dead. The first thing she said was, 'I feel so good. Am I alive?' "

Added Lown: "Consider this: administering the parade of anti-arrhythmic drugs took five hours and her cardiac function actually deteriorated as a result of these drugs. By contrast, use of synchronized countershock required but a few minutes of preparation, reversion was instantaneous, and there were no evident side effects."

That procedure at the Peter Bent Brigham and numerous procedures like it performed at other hospitals during the same period were the last act of the first age of arrhythmia research, the culmination of all that electrophysiology had accomplished in two hundred years of experimentation and investigation. Electroshock was finally consistently saving lives. It took two centuries, but fulfilled at last were the hopes of all the early eighteenth-century Humane Societies whose mandate was to promote the then radical concept that electricity could be used to resuscitate "persons apparently dead."

With the closing of the first age of arrhythmia research, its modern era began serendipitously three years later in a laboratory at New York's Columbia-Presbyterian Hospital, when on a September day an entirely accidental electrophysiological breakthrough occurred during a routine procedure. It was one of those unexpected research anomalies so common in medical literature as a prelude to sudden shifts in clinical thought — and with it the boundaries stifling electrophysiology were effectively demolished.

It is not hyperbole to say that that day at Columbia-Presbyterian electrophysiology merged with cardiology, though only in hindsight is this apparent. It would be the mid-1980s before the discipline growing out of this merger would have more than a tiny cadre of physicians (cardiologists who are still today considered part of a medical avant-garde) in its fold. Indeed, while the operation was proceeding at Columbia-Presbyterian, these new cardiologists were barely teenagers.

Thomas Bigger, a cardiologist at Columbia-Presbyterian, was a medical tyro in 1965, a thirty-year-old research fellow at the hospital, putting in the usual sixty-hour weeks making rounds, at times not sleeping or breathing fresh outdoor air for three days at a clip. Bigger was training with Dr. Brian Hoffman in cellular electrophysiology. He was impaling single cells with microscopic glass tubes to analyze the electrical functions of these organisms through their fluids, but he couldn't quiet the urge to apply electrophysiology to patients, an urge that had been instilled a few years earlier by Gordon Moe. Though Bigger had not yet met Moe, as a medical student in the late 1950s at the Medical College of Georgia, he had avidly followed Moe's activities in papers and at medical symposia and was convinced that his mentor-at-a-distance was on to something significant.

What most interested Bigger was Moe's tenacious laboratory research into the atrioventricular nodes of dogs. The A-V node, where the atria and the ventricles meet, is second in importance as a cardiac electrical stimulating center only to the sinoatrial node, the heart's primary pacemaker. Moe's intention in studying canine hearts was to unearth the particular qualities of the A-V node. His aim was to detail how the A-V node spreads its complex electrical cadence to the ventricles and to diagram the role that the autonomic nervous system, which has a direct line to the A-V node, plays in initiating and choreographing heart rhythms.

Bigger, a Georgian with a soft, slow-paced Southern cadence in his voice, is a man with a churning curiosity. A researcher who rejects unwarranted experimentation on human beings, Bigger is also an activist who cannot abide medical foot-dragging. So by the mid-1960s, Bigger had decided that electrophysiology was moving too slowly. It was time, he believed, to take Moe's work with animals one radical step farther. Consequently, he opted to investigate the A-V node in human beings.

To do this, he transformed Columbia-Presbyterian's cath lab, where thin tubes called catheters were inserted into patients' hearts for diagnostic purposes, into the first full-fledged cardiac electrophysiology center at a major hospital in the United States.

Part of my regular routine was doing cardiac catheterization procedures two days a week in the lab. I got pretty proficient at these and I was able to complete my work quickly, so I started thinking, "As long as I have the patient here anyway, perhaps we could do some electrical stimulation sequences in human beings and see how people's A-V nodes operate." Understanding the human A-V node better was what I was after. It was only an extension of Gordon Moe's work with animals — and also that of my mentor at the hospital, Brian Hoffman.

What Bigger was after and what he got were clearly two different things. One day in September 1965, a twenty-one-year-old man was brought into the cath lab for evaluation of an enlarged heart, a cardiac abnormality that had been present since birth.

The catheterization took thirty-five minutes, but I had the lab booked for over an hour if I needed it. So, with a half an hour to spend, I started studying the patient's A-V node function by delivering programmed electrical stimuli to the patient's atria and observing the responses. Lo and behold, somehow his heart became arrhythmic completely out of the blue.

We immediately were able to stop the arrhythmia with the stimulator. But then I wondered, did I start that arrhythmia myself? Gordon Moe in all his years of working with dogs had only one animal in which an arrhythmia started unexpectedly in his laboratory. And then he was never able to do it again. So we tested whether we were in control of this patient's arrhythmia or whether it was pure coincidence that it occurred when it did. We attempted to start and stop it by delivering well-timed electrical stimuli. It worked! We were actually able to turn this patient's arrhythmia on and off at will.

Bigger is unable to hide his self-satisfaction when he speaks of that day. It is the ultimate conceit of a physician to be able to control the physiology of life. There is hubris in all doctors that says, if I have to lose to death so often, then at least once give me the opportunity to manipulate the systems of life. And that's exactly what Bigger did: he had created a cardiac arrhythmia where there was none before. To an electrophysiologist, this was akin to delivering a baby from a woman who isn't pregnant.

Of course, to carry this analogy further, Bigger's patient *was* pregnant, it just wasn't showing.

Bigger had recorded the entire cath lab event with an electrocardiograph and intracardiac electrograms. So, after studying the EKG and asking the young patient a lot of questions about his medical history and how his heart had reacted in different circumstances throughout his life, Bigger knew that the twenty-one-year-old had been suffering bouts of tachycardia since he was born. These arrhythmias were supraventricular — that is, located in the atria, not the ventricles — and were thus not life threatening like the more deadly ventricular arrhythmias. The young man's arrhythmias had never been diagnosed before, mainly because of general ignorance about the condition among most physicians.

I understood immediately why Moe had only once been able to induce an arrhythmia in the laboratory on his dogs. If a patient doesn't have a propensity to arrhythmias you won't be able to stimulate one. Apparently none of Moe's dogs except the one in which he induced an arrhythmia had an underlying arrhythmic heart. I was fortunate to come upon a patient that day who was born with a situation that made him prone to arrhythmias.

Bigger realized that he had hit upon something important. So he began to experiment on one or two patients a week who had a history of arrhythmias to see if he could at will start and stop supraventricular tachycardia and to determine the exact mechanism for doing this. Slowly and steadily the data built up. Before long it became clear that patients with spontaneous supraventricular arrhythmias were indeed inducible in the laboratory in most cases, if the electrical stimuli that precipitated them were timed correctly.

To Bigger, this period of experimentation was painfully deliberate. The pace of it was not to his liking. He felt it threatened to hinder and dilute the impact of his breakthrough in the cath lab.

After we first induced an arrhythmia that day, we were impatient to find out whether arrhythmias could be started in all patients who had already suffered tachycardias. Remember, up until then we only had one dog and one person and we wanted more information quickly. But Columbia-Presbyterian is a conservative institution. And these studies required me to put catheters in the right side of the heart, still somewhat radical fare during the 1960s. So recruiting subjects and amassing a lot of data for this was pretty slow going.

While the conservatism of Columbia-Presbyterian impeded Bigger, the hospital's growing reputation for breakthroughs in electrophysiological research buttressed him. It was there, for instance, that André Cournand and Dickinson Richards conducted landmark research that resulted in successful electrical measurements of the heart through catheters — and won the Nobel Prize for this experimentation in 1957. The support of this faction at the hospital encouraged Bigger to continue, even when patient enrollment in his research was slow.

Over time more and more data accrued, until the physiology of how consistently to repeat his 1965 cath lab "accident" became clear to him. Unmasking the properties of supraventricular arrhythmias was an intensive effort. It was not unlike putting together tiles of different shapes and sizes so that all the seams are hidden and the pattern is flawless. But when he had finished the floor plan for his model of how a cardiac arrhythmia is started and stopped, the pieces meshed perfectly.

Bigger learned that if a series of equally spaced electrical pulses are delivered to the atria at a rate faster than their intrinsic heartbeat, the cardiac rhythm shifts gears and takes on the more rapid cadence of the new, quicker pulse. Then, if a premature stimulus is added to this rapidly beating heart, various regions of the heart react quite differently. Some are slow to recover from the heartbeat and some recover quickly, depending on their intrinsic electrical properties and how healthy the cells are. Areas in the heart that are slow to recover may serve as conduction barriers to subsequent premature electrical stimuli and cause enough local electrical disturbance to result in extra bursts known as echo beats or extrasystoles. At times, this arrhythmic cadence may become repetitive and throw the heart into rapid heart rhythm known as tachycardia.

And with this elegant but complex explanation, not only had Bigger and his associate at the time, Dr. Bruce Goldreyer, deduced the recipe for starting an arrhythmia in the clinical environment, they also had replicated the very blueprint that the body itself uses for precipitating some arrhythmias.

Finally, in 1970, Bigger and Goldreyer published their preliminary findings on how the commonest form of supraventricular arrhythmias work. They immediately received independent confirmation that their approach was correct. Unbeknown to Bigger, a French cardiologist, Phillipe Coumel, was performing exactly the same experimentation on patients in Paris and had come up with the same model for supraventricular arrhythmias.

In hindsight, Bigger admits that he was fortunate to have achieved his unexpected cath lab breakthrough on a patient who had a supraventricular arrhythmia — an arrhythmia of the upper chambers of the heart or atria — precisely because these are frequently not life threatening, unlike the potentially deadly ventricular arrhythmias.

The reason that atrial arrhythmias are benign is simple: the normal atrial pulse is seventy to eighty beats per minute, a sufficient output to excite the ventricles into pumping efficiently. Even if the atrial rhythm becomes very rapid, however, the ventricles pump in normal cadence and sequence, albeit rapidly, after each atrial contraction, thereby allowing adequate filling of the ventricles and preserving in most instances the proper performance of the heart. Furthermore, most supraventricular tachycardias occur in otherwise healthy people without heart disease. Because of this, supraventricular tachy-cardias usually are not life threatening, even though they may cause severely discomforting symptoms; on the other hand, ventricular tachycardias usually signal cardiac disease. As many as one in every thirty Americans has supraventricular arrhyth-mias, and most likely will never know or suffer any ill-health from them.

Because we were only inducing supraventricular tachy-cardias during our experimentation, we could explore without fear. We knew that we could revert the arrhythmia without any damage to the patient. But had we achieved this breakthrough with a patient who had a ventricular arrhythmia, we might have made a lot of mistakes and killed a lot of people. It's even possible that we would never have gotten as far as we did. But this work with supraventricular arrhythmias, where we could afford to explore its characteristics without fear, fully served as the model for evaluation of more deadly ventricular rhythms later.

Bigger's research was a medical landmark, but it wasn't until the late 1970s that clinical electrophysiology was recognized as the springboard for a new medical discipline. By that point, those future electrophysiologists who were teenagers in 1965 had grown up, completed medical school, and were in their own hospital research laboratories. Individually, they were a radical lot for physicians, enamored with the possibilities of new medical techniques. Some dabbled with computers. Others designed innovative cardiac devices. Still others worked to overhaul the very concept of emergency cardiac medicine. As a group, nevertheless, they were homogeneous. Their narrow purpose was finally to put clinical electrophysiology on the map. In the end, they were to create a series of investigative, di-agnostic, and treatment strategies that would save the lives of many of those previously doomed to sudden death.

·4·

Testing the Limits of
Sudden Cardiac Death

MEDICAL revolutions occur because many minds share the same goal and thoughts. Though propelled by individuals, they are group efforts that leapfrog from one research unit to another, with each staking claims in more and more difficult clinical territories. The growth of clinical electrophysiology is an example of such a revolution. And one of the many researchers who have ensured the emergence of electrophysiology is Jeremy Ruskin, director of the Cardiac Arrhythmia Service at Massachusetts General Hospital.

Ruskin graduated from Harvard Medical School in 1971 and completed his training in internal medicine in 1973. That year, as a result of the advice and influence of one of his clinical teachers, Ruskin went to study with Anthony Damato at the United States Public Health Service Hospital on Staten Island. Damato's small electrophysiological research unit had a worldwide reputation and attracted many of today's brightest clinical electrophysiologists. Those who would go on to found arrhythmia research centers at — besides Massachusetts General — the University of Illinois, the University of Pennsylvania, Duke

University, and Milwaukee's Mount Sinai Hospital, to name just a few, met and exchanged ideas under the disciplined tutelage of Damato.

To become involved in arrhythmia research was a risky path for those who chose it at that stage. There were so many highly publicized breakthroughs and success stories in other areas of cardiology then that it was extremely tempting for any young physician to follow the better-traveled roads to quick glory and not get involved in a more esoteric, perhaps fruitless, subspeciality like electrophysiology. The growth of coronary angiography — X rays that provide detailed, intracardiac pictures of how vessels to the heart are performing in real time — as well as other imaging techniques, was offering mainstream cardiology microscopically precise investigative tools for diagnosing failed and clogged blood lines. With the most intimate functions of a patient's cardiac region so accurately depicted by the angiogram, therapeutic solutions for arterial blockage such as bypass grafting and balloon angioplasty evolved rapidly. No such dramatic and lucrative interventions accompanied the early development of clinical electrophysiology. Says Jeremy Ruskin:

In the early 1970s there was a period of extraordinarily rapid growth in modern, invasive cardiology that was much more dramatic, much more rewarding, and much less speculative than arrhythmia research, which was not considered a highly practical branch of cardiology then. Most people entering cardiology when I did preferred to learn about hemodynamics, angiography, and imaging rather than electrophysiology. But my experience at Tony Damato's lab was such a revelation and so exciting that I never had second thoughts about not pursuing clinical research in some other aspect of cardiology. What I saw in that lab was an opportunity to do both investigative and clinical work at the same time, using new and powerful technologies as tools.

Basically, what was being studied at the Public Health Service on Staten Island through the mid-1970s were supraventricular tachycardias and the physiology of the conduction system of the heart — much of the same research matter that had occupied clinical electrophysiologists for several years. In many ways, electrophysiology was at something of a standstill. Inducing benign supraventricular arrhythmias in susceptible patients, once a seemingly unobtainable achievement, was relatively easy and trouble-proof. Clinical electrophysiologists took it for granted, the way most of us reacted to man's ability to explore and survive on the moon during that period. But moving to the next guidepost in electrophysiology, to examine deadly human ventricular arrhythmias — to turn them on and off at will in the laboratory — required a leap of clinical acumen and an equal leap in courage that seemed daunting.

At the time that I was in Staten Island, ventricular arrhythmias were still viewed with a great deal of fear, in that we really had very little idea of what we were dealing with or how they worked. Electrical instability in the ventricle was thought to be associated with the risk of sudden death. So we were very hesitant to do anything to a patient that might provoke ventricular tachycardia or ventricular fibrillation and perhaps kill him.

It wasn't until 1975, when Ruskin had finished his work on Staten Island and moved to Massachusetts General Hospital, that he and others began tackling the problem of sudden cardiac death. The impetus, Ruskin says, was simple: it became apparent that ventricular arrhythmias represented a significant public health danger. Hundreds of thousands of people were dying each year from ventricular arrhythmias, people who were alive, even vigorous, one second and dead the next without warning. Indeed, even those few patients fortunate enough to be snatched from the grip of death and resuscitated during a critical arrhythmic event were just being sent back to their homes, essentially untreated; up to 40 percent of them would have another bout with sudden death during the next twelve to twenty-four months. The chances of their surviving this second life-threatening incident were slim. Nothing less than fresh ideas and aggressive research was necessary to solve this problem.

One of the first to ambitiously research sudden cardiac death and the use of electrophysiological techniques in patients with ventricular tachycardia was the Dutch physician Dr. Hein Wellens. Wellens found that arrhythmias could frequently be reproduced and terminated in these patients using carefully timed electrical stimuli delivered to the ventricles through a catheter. A few years later, Dr. Mark Josephson and his colleagues at the University of Pennsylvania confirmed and expanded these observations and carried out pioneering research on the mechanisms of ventricular tachycardia.

The studies of Wellens and Josephson supported the concept that the commonest form of ventricular tachycardia, that occurring in patients with disease of the coronary arteries, resulted from an abnormality known as reentry — a repetitive movement of electricity over an abnormal pathway or circuit in the ventricles. Critical insights such as this into the mechanisms of ventricular arrhythmias and the new-found ability to start and stop some forms of ventricular tachycardia in the controlled environment of a clinical laboratory that emerged with these insights intrigued Ruskin.

And in the late 1970s, Ruskin and his associate, Hasan Garan, began conducting similar studies on patients who had been successfully resuscitated from an episode of cardiac arrest. Garan arrived at Massachusetts General as a Cardiac Fellow with a strong background in physiology not long after Ruskin began his research at the hospital. While training in the basics of cardiology, Garan grew increasingly interested in electrophysiology and started working with Ruskin. When his fellowship was over, Garan stayed on at MGH as codirector of the Arrhythmia Service.

In their initial research, Ruskin and Garan identified thirty-one patients who had collapsed suddenly and unexpectedly of ventricular arrhythmias. Following resuscitation and recovery, these patients were temporarily in stable condition but were known to be at extremely high risk for another potentially fatal cardiac arrest.

The patients were observed in an intensive care unit while their use of anti-arrhythmic drugs was discontinued for several days. Massachusetts General clinicians then inserted a series of electrode catheters into veins in the thigh and arm. Monitored through a fluoroscope, the electrodes were positioned at several different sites within the heart. A variety of programmed electrical pulses was then delivered through the catheters to the heart in an attempt to provoke ventricular arrhythmias.

Ruskin and Garan's efforts were rewarded. Ventricular arrhythmias were induced in twenty-five of the thirty-one patients. (Of the six other patients, two had ventricular arrhythmias that, ironically, could only be induced when they were taking anti-arrhythmic drugs; in the four additional cases, either no cardiac rhythm abnormalities were found upon further testing or the patient had an atrial and not a ventricular arrhythmia.) The induced ventricular arrhythmias were quickly stopped with countershocks, returning the heart rhythm to normal in all patients.

This experiment and others like it occurring across the country at the same time were watersheds in both electrophysiology and cardiology. It was an important precursor to the success stories coming out of hospital arrhythmia units today. Cardiologists were finally face to face with the deadly ventricular arrhythmia on their terms. Because they could at last turn a ventricular arrhythmia on and off at will by provoking and defusing it with an artificial, man-made stimulus, cardiologists could now examine the ventricular arrhythmia in its environment and as it occurred, the first step to understanding it and ultimately disabling it with drugs or other forms of therapy.

Most important, electrophysiologists finally could design clinical strategies to counter the fruitless methods previously used to treat patients who survived cardiac arrest. Heart disease is a complex condition but, in many cases, performing surgery on coronary arteries or on cardiac valves while ignoring the underlying arrhythmias is like seeing a patient with severe emphysema and a bloody nose, merely stopping the nose bleed, and pronouncing the patient cured. The other condition, the one that will probably be fatal before long, is left to continue to do its damage.

The first clinical strategy that emerged from the ability to induce ventricular arrhythmias in the cath lab is a reworking of an old technique that had failed patients time after time: the random use of anti-arrhythmic drugs. If a patient's condition has not reached the critical stage, it is often desirable to use noninvasive treatment with drugs that stabilize the electrical system of the heart. And while few electrophysiologists disagree with this approach, the double edge of this protocol — the way the drugs react quite differently from one patient to the next and the fact that they sometimes provoke and exacerbate life-threatening arrhythmias instead of preventing them — has made anti-arrhythmic drug treatment something of a clinical pariah.

But now that ventricular arrhythmias can be started and stopped in the laboratory, electrophysiologists are able, with trial and error, to test the efficacy and safety of anti-arrhythmic drugs before sending a patient home with a bottle of pills. First, a drug — perhaps quinidine or procainamide — is administered to the patient for several days, and then electrical stimulation of the heart is repeated in an attempt to make the ventricular arrhythmia recur in the cath lab. If no sign of ventricular tachycardia or fibrillation appears, the drug is considered adequate. But if a ventricular arrhythmia ensues, alternative medications are assessed in the cath lab until an adequate drug regimen is found.

This trial-and-error procedure is significant. It breaks the vicious cycle that a patient can suffer for years as drug after drug fails and a drastically diminished quality of life is a result of the side effects and the inefficacy of randomly prescribed combinations of toxic pharmaceuticals.

Too often — in at least one-third of all patients treated by electrophysiologists — drugs are still not the solution for cardiac arrhythmias. The erratic behavior of anti-arrhythmia drugs simply rules them out as a final, acceptable clinical choice. In those many cases where drugs are not a desirable alternative, such options as anti-arrhythmia surgery and the implantation of an automatic defibrillator to prevent or terminate the arrhythmia when it occurs are used.

The decision as to which anti-arrhythmia therapy to choose is a difficult one. There are no predefined formulas for treating an arrhythmia patient. Unlike most other clinical disciplines or subdisciplines, every arrhythmia patient is a unique case requiring vastly different medical strategies. Says Ruskin:

> An appropriate approach to an arrhythmia requires sorting through many patient variables and an increasingly wide range of treatment options. The goal is to evaluate each patient's situation in sufficient detail to allow one to devise, with the patient's participation, a therapeutic approach that is best suited to that individual's needs.
>
> The process is demanding and time consuming. It requires a lifetime of experience and the use of intelligence and creativity to select the correct arrhythmia therapy.

All of these treatment options, though, rely on one central medical concept that grew out of the ventricular arrhythmia research of the small core of investigators around the country in the 1970s and early 1980s: if you can induce a ventricular arrhythmia and actually watch it swell from a potential cardiac electrical malfunction to a kinetic one, you can study its mechanism, test the safety and effectiveness of drugs in preventing its occurrence, and sometimes even pinpoint its exact location in the heart. Then, with the arrhythmia's characteristics and behavior defined, specific therapy, whether it be drugs, surgery, an implantable defibrillator, or a combination of these can be selected to meet each patient's unique needs. Adds Ruskin:

The treatment of cardiac arrhythmias at Massachusetts General and other centers that specialize in this problem is a very complicated one because of the large number of relatively new therapeutic options that have recently become available. In many ways, these new approaches constitute an embarrassment of riches, compared to what was available to patients only a few years ago.

·5·

Basement Notes from the Bulfinch: The Case of Margaret W.

I N the Massachusetts General Hospital's Bulfinch basement, where the offices of Jeremy Ruskin's Cardiac Arrhythmia Service are located, the ceilings are low; the maze of peeling pipes overhead hang down almost to eye level and sweat hot, steamy air even in the warmest days of summer. The cement walls separating the narrowest of walkways are painted in concrete-bunker tones of off-green and farther-off beige. Only the climate-controlled physicians' offices that line the tightly knit corridors depart from the prevailing institutional gloom. And then only barely so.

The design of Ruskin's office, like that of others in the Bulfinch's lower level, attempts — in vain — to cosmeticize the charmless basement. The wood paneling and shelving on masonry walls, the oak desk, and carpeted concrete floor fail to camouflage the thick pipes on the ceiling. Underground, after all, is underground.

To Ruskin, though, the location and decor of his office are trivial matters about which he thinks little. As he darts down the Bulfinch basement hallways toward the electrophysiology lab, he prepares himself, running through the clinical history of the patient he's about to treat in the lab; recalling what he knows about the arrhythmia; and concentrating on those concepts about the case that will be central to the upcoming procedure.

The most important issues relate to the type of arrhythmia that is being treated — its mechanism and location in the heart. It's also important to know as much as possible about the structural anatomy of each patient's heart: are there any abnormalities of the coronary arteries which supply blood to the heart; is the heart muscle damaged; are there abnormalities of any of the heart valves and, if so, what is the cause? These anatomic and structural components of the heart are central to the way the heart functions. In particular, the degree to which they affect the capacity of the heart muscle to pump efficiently is one of the most critical determinants of long-term survival for arrhythmia patients and influences in an important way the kinds of therapeutic alternatives that are available to them.

Like most things in medicine, the most successful arrhythmia therapy is highly individualized. Each patient's problem has unique features and responds differently to various clinical interventions. The evaluation and rational treatment of cardiac arrhythmias is a time-consuming and demanding process, which must take into account a number of factors, including the structural anatomy of the heart, the detailed characteristics of the arrhythmia itself, the patient's age and general physical condition, and the patient's psychological makeup and personal preferences.

When Ruskin arrives at the electrophysiology lab this morning, his patient, Margaret W., is already on the operating table; covered with green hospital sheets, she looks calmly at the ceiling, locked in her own thoughts as physicians and a technician prepare the catheters and electrical instrumentation that will support her anti-arrhythmia procedure. In the outer room of the lab, on the other side of a glass wall from the patient and staff, Ruskin puts on a heavy lead apron to shield himself from X rays.

The electrophysiology lab itself is crowded, both with people and machines. A tiny room, only twelve feet by twenty feet, it is difficult to move about in without tripping over bulky wiring or stepping on toes. On one wall is an array of cardiac recording equipment that monitors every blip and pulse of the patient's heartbeat. Next to this is a stimulation device that the electrode catheters, which will be positioned in the patient's heart, are attached to. The catheters will stimulate the patient's heart into its incipient arrhythmia.

Looming over the patient are the heavy "eye" and arms of a fluoroscope, the X-ray device that will track the progress of the catheters until they reach the correct location in the heart. The fluoroscope screen, on which the black-and-white image of the heart will be displayed, is located near the patient's table.

Adjacent to the fluoroscope is a round metal paddle — six inches in diameter, it looks like a gleaming, silver mutant lollypop — which is connected to a defibrillator, a machine with switches and dials at the ready to countershock the patient out of tachycardia or fibrillation.

Margaret W. is unmoved by the activity around her and the machines. The fifty-four-year-old woman has suffered through a lifetime of rheumatic heart disease and has lived for the past six years with a persistent atrial arrhythmia that has incapacitated her. Finally, Ruskin has offered her a way out of her medical problems. A religious and optimistic woman, she is resolved and sanguine about a successful outcome.

Margaret W.'s problems began with rheumatic fever, which she developed as a teenager. Over a period of many years, this led to chronic rheumatic heart disease, which slowly destroyed two of the most important structures in her heart, the aortic and mitral valves.

The mitral valve is located between the left atrium, which receives oxygenated blood from the lungs, and the left ventricle. The mitral valve allows blood to flow from the upper chamber into the lower chamber and not the other way.

The aortic valve lies between the main pumping chamber of the heart, the left ventricle, and the aorta, the heart's largest artery and the vessel that carries oxygenated blood to the vital organs and the rest of the body. When the aortic valve opens, blood is allowed to enter the aorta; when it closes, it ensures that blood does not leak back into the left ventricle.

As a result of rheumatic heart disease, Margaret W.'s aortic and mitral valves became thickened, scarred, and nonpliable. Because they neither opened nor closed properly, they impeded blood flow in the normal directions; they also leaked.

In 1981, medical technology caught up with Margaret W.'s condition, and both her mitral and aortic valves were replaced with prosthetic valves. Initially, Margaret W. had an excellent result from her surgery. Her valve problems were relieved — there were no further obstructions or leaks and the flow of blood in her heart was returned to normal. However, within a short time, she began to experience a variety of arrhythmias, including atrial tachycardia, atrial flutter, and atrial fibrillation.

These arrhythmias resulted from severe scarring and enlargement of the atria, a common long-term consequence of chronic rheumatic heart disease and one that frequently disrupts the electrical system of the heart. Consequently, despite the fact that Margaret W.'s ventricles were unscathed and her artificial valves were functioning normally, she suffered almost incessant tachycardias, a rapid pulse of up to 180 beats per minute, which left her weak, short of breath, and entirely unable to exert herself.

Soon after her surgery in 1981, Margaret W. was admitted to a medical center in Boston where anti-arrhythmia drugs were prescribed. She was treated with the gamut of all available anti-arrhythmic drugs, singly and in multiple combinations — enough to make her sick — and none solved her problem. Finally, after five years of battling the side effects of drugs as well as her incapacitating arrhythmias, she was referred to Massachusetts General Hospital.

Ruskin examined Margaret W. in late 1986 and concluded

that her atrial arrhythmias could not be stopped, but recommended that they be eliminated by destroying the tissue through which they were conducted to the ventricles. Essentially, Ruskin's decision was to let the ventricles make their own pace, ignoring the atrium. In short, shut down the primary power system and let the equally adequate backup system take over at a slower and more comfortable rate.

This procedure is known among electrophysiologists as inducing A-V, or atrioventricular block. The goal is to interrupt electrical communication between the atrium and ventricles at the bundle of His, a critical point in the heart's wiring system at which the atria are electrically coupled to the ventricles.

In this particular situation, A-V block is created by delivering an electrical shock to the bundle of His through a special electrode catheter that is inserted into a vein and guided into a precise position within the heart. This revolutionary technique in arrhythmia therapy, known as *transcatheter electrical ablation,* was first performed by Dr. Melvin Scheinman at the University of California in San Francisco and is now being refined and used at a small number of arrhythmia centers around the world.

Entering the electrophysiology lab quietly, Ruskin nods at the physicians and technicians and walks over to Margaret W. He touches her brow.

"Mrs. W., are you okay? We're ready to go."

She answers calmly. Her eyes move toward Ruskin, but her face remains pointed, unwaveringly and determinedly, at the ceiling.

"I'm fine. And ready."

There's a quiet, unspoken tension in the room. Two other physicians and a technician are at their places: one about to man the catheters, another positioning the fluoroscope directly over the patient's heart, and the third ready to operate the bank of cardiac stimulation and monitoring devices.

A thin, Teflon-coated electrode catheter is inserted into Margaret W.'s femoral vein. The patient hardly moves as the catheter enters her body; numbed by a local anesthetic, she experiences the small incision as nothing more than a pinprick.

The fluoroscope is turned on. On its monitor is the X-ray image of Margaret W.'s heart; the metal and plastic valves are clearly discernible — they look like tiny gates in a pinball machine, opening as the blood pulses through them and then closing tightly when the cardiac chamber is emptied. Ruskin stares at the fluoroscope screen for a few seconds, watching the valves, deep in thought, then walks over to the bank of cardiac monitors. The senior lab technician, Charles Freeman, points to an LED readout and says, "Her heart rate is varying between 140 and 160 most of the time, though I've had a reading or two as high as 180."

The catheter is moved slowly toward Margaret W.'s heart; the operating physician looks as if he's alternately tightening and loosening a screw as he snakes the catheter carefully up into the patient's body. Finally, the very tip of the catheter appears on the fluoroscope screen, near the center of the heart.

Ruskin walks back over to the fluoroscope screen, pausing on his way to look at his patient and ask if she's all right.

"I'm fine. I don't feel a thing."

"You're doing great."

Ruskin answers her almost absentmindedly as he stares at the fluoroscope monitor. More of the catheter has reached Margaret W.'s heart, but it is still in the right atrium, a few inches above its target in the bundle of His, where the right atrium and right ventricles meet.

"Move that catheter down, if you can," Ruskin suggests.

The clockwise then counterclockwise movements of the catheter continue as the operating physician tries to position it in the heart. A look of frustration covers his face. "The catheter is not cooperating."

"I don't think that you're going to make it with this one," Ruskin responds, still staring at the screen and the wayward catheter. "Try another catheter."

In the midst of all of this, Margaret W. remains impassive and unmoved. She seems to have distanced herself from the procedure as if she is watching somebody else lying on the patient's table. Meanwhile a new catheter has been positioned in Margaret W.'s heart. Ruskin continues to prowl from machine to machine. It is a curious brand of medicine that he and his colleagues practice. Physicians used to rely on information coursing from their soft, knowledgeable hands for diagnoses and treatments; now they depend on microchips to analyze onrushing data pouring out of wires and electrodes.

This time the catheter is moving correctly toward its target, the bundle of His. Ruskin turns to Freeman.

"It's OK to call anesthesia. We're just about ready."

Ruskin gazes quietly at the fluoroscope monitor, watching the catheter as it seats gently against the bundle of His. Then he says, to no one in particular, thinking out loud, "Those prosthetic valves are operating so smoothly, aren't they?" He is clearly worried, though, and walks out into the laboratory's anteroom to wait for the anesthesiologist.

Her prosthetic valves really concern me. We're about to send a significant jolt of electricity into her heart right next to where those valves are seated. I'm worried about the possibility of damaging one or both of her prosthetic valves with the shock.

Back in the lab, with the anesthesiologist present, Ruskin walks over to the cardiac monitors. "We're getting an excellent recording from the bundle of His," says Freeman. "The catheter is placed perfectly and it's stable. We're ready to deliver the shock."

Ruskin leans over Margaret W.

"The anesthesiologist is going to give you some medications which will make you sleep for about five minutes. Everything is going well. When you wake up, you should feel quite a bit better."

Margaret W. nods slowly. The first glimmer of tension crosses her face as the anesthesiologist begins to place the mask over her mouth and nose.

"Dr. Ruskin, do me a favor, tell my sisters as soon as you know that I'm okay. They worry about me."

"Absolutely."

Within sixty seconds, Margaret W. is unconscious. Ruskin places the silver defibrillator paddle on her chest and nods to the technician at the bank of cardiac monitors. A dial is turned, a button is pushed, and a 50-joule shock is shot into the bundle of His of Margaret W.'s heart. (A joule is a unit of energy equal to ten million ergs that is used to define the working output of electroshock devices.) Margaret W.'s body bends sharply forward as her chest muscles contract with the force of the electroshock.

Ruskin quickly looks over at the readout of her heartbeat. As the electroshock subsides, in an abrupt shift the digital display of Margaret W.'s heartbeat changes from 143 one moment to a comfortable, safe 60 the next. The heart block is successful. The atrial arrhythmia is no longer being conducted to the ventricles. A far more manageable electrical rhythm, known as a junctional rhythm (originating in the junction between the atria and ventricles) is setting the pace of her cardiac pumping chambers.

Ruskin darts over to the fluoroscope monitor, examining the prosthetic valves carefully. They are still intact and do not appear to have been disrupted by the shock, for they continue to open and close smoothly.

A smile crosses Ruskin's face and the mood in the lab shifts noticeably. The physicians and technician begin to remove the catheter from Margaret W.'s body and unhook her from the ganglia of wires to which she is attached. For the first time, now that this difficult procedure has been a success, the other physicians and Ruskin start chatting among themselves, indulging in topical humor. Jokes about the Iran-Contra debacle, Oliver North, Fawn Hall, and Robert McFarlane — real-world boondoggles of human greed and error, not life-and-death clinical concerns — erase the tension in the room.

Slowly, Margaret W. wakes up. She smiles broadly as she feels the slow pace of her heart. Her gray, tired-looking skin seems rejuvenated; it is now a pulsating pink.

"I haven't felt this good in years. I thought I'd never feel this good again. I feel as though I could get up and walk out of here."

Ruskin walks over to her, takes her hand, and pats it.

"Your heartbeat is averaging about 70 — half of what it was before this procedure. At times it is even down to 60."

"Tell my sisters."

Seventy-two hours later, Margaret W. will walk out of Massachusetts General with a small pacemaker, implanted in a subsequent procedure, and a heartbeat even more normal and unwavering than most of us have, no longer crippled by shortness of breath or fatigue. As Ruskin puts it, "Her life won't be controlled any longer by her arrhythmia."

Back in his office, Ruskin is noticeably relaxed. Tired, but enjoying the pleasure of a successful outcome for a few moments, Ruskin remarks that although he and his colleagues have performed many procedures like these, they still seem remarkable, almost otherworldly in their ability to affect a damaged heart so poignantly. It strikes him as impressive that closed chest surgery, utilizing only the tip of a catheter skitted in through a tiny pinhole in the body, could have such an marked impact on a patient's condition and quality of life.

Just a few years ago, open heart surgery was required to create atrioventricular block. It was a major procedure with some risk and significant postoperative discomfort for the patient. The beauty of these kinds of catheter procedures is that they accomplish the same goals as surgery but are less invasive. They attempt to intervene directly at the site responsible for the arrhythmia, without disturbing other areas of the heart and without a major surgical incision and prolonged general anesthesia. These techniques are still in the process of being developed and refined, but they hold enormous promise for the treatment of some patients with arrhythmias.

·6·

The Ether Dome

O F the more than two thousand hospitals across the country, fewer than 3 percent have cardiac arrhythmia units. Sites specializing in treating sudden cardiac arrest using the clinical wisdom amassed over two centuries by electrophysiologists are still quite uncommon in the nation's health care delivery system. Despite the fact that resistance to electrophysiology by physicians has softened greatly in recent years, in many hospitals the sheer anachronistic muscle of old-line, mainstream cardiologists and traditional cardiological thought continues to work against the founding of arrhythmia units.

The Arrhythmia Service at Massachusetts General is now recognized as one of the jewels of the sudden cardiac death centers in the United States. But its presence at the hospital, like the existence of virtually all arrhythmia units, is not an anomaly or an accident or a simple tribute to current clinical trends. Rather it is the result of the fortuitous interlacing at Massachusetts General of three unique historical and modern-day factors: for one, Massachusetts General has a tradition of being a starkly forward-thinking hospital, a site where clinical barriers have been, and still are, broken frequently; for another, cardiology and advanced heart research were literally invented at MGH; and thirdly, the Arrhythmia Service was fostered by an extremely creative management direction set by the head of the Cardiology Unit that nourished and favored the most challenging clinical and research efforts.

At first blush it could be said that the Arrhythmia Service at Massachusetts General was founded by necessity and default. When Jeremy Ruskin and Hasan Garan instituted it in 1977, they had just completed the experiments in which they induced potentially fatal arrhythmias in controlled laboratory conditions and then as successfully shut them down. Word had spread quickly through the medical community of this and other clinical procedures Ruskin, his team, and others at a small number of centers around the country were developing to thwart future episodes of tachycardia and fibrillation among patients who had "died" and been resuscitated. Before long, an increasing number of cardiologists — some still skeptical of electrophysiology — began to refer their essentially terminal patients to Ruskin and Garan. And as the patient load grew, it became clear to some administrators at MGH that a full-fledged Arrhythmia Service was needed.

But the Arrhythmia Service would never have survived and prospered had it not been fervently championed from the very start by Edgar Haber, then chief of cardiology at Massachusetts General. Even when other physicians were taking a wait-and-see stance, Haber threw his whole-hearted support behind Ruskin and Garan's research. Haber's endorsement of the electrophysiologists was not surprising. As an administrator and a leading basic scientist, Haber, who left Massachusetts General in 1988 to become a research director for a pharmaceutical firm, cut his own path and ignored trendy rules of management. Unlike many other leaders in academic medicine these days, Haber is medically eclectic. Bucking the one-track staffing formulas that many hospital chiefs subscribe to, he made it a policy to recruit physicians for his department who are involved in all areas of cardiology; in the process, Haber strengthened without bias every aspect of clinical and investigative cardiology at Massachusetts General.

Haber's cardiology department seemed to make good medical sense, but in the widely divergent clinical leanings of its physicians it runs counter to the way in which many hospitals are staffed in this age of specialization. It's chic these days for hospital managers, both in the for-profit or in the equally cutthroat, not-for-profit markets, to stress their department's or institution's expertise in substrata of medical care — be it an aspect of surgery, bioresearch, or organ transplantation, among many other possibilities.

The Memorial Sloan-Kettering Cancer Center in New York City is a good example. Paul Marks became president of Sloan-Kettering in 1980, at a time when it was competing feverishly for funds with other not-for-profit institutions in the New York metropolitan area and losing out frequently. In order to succeed in the big donation wars, Marks let it be known, nearly from the day of his appointment, that Sloan-Kettering was no longer a typical "generalist" surgical cancer center but instead would primarily attack cancer through research, specifically in molecular biology. Physicians and surgeons whose backgrounds didn't fit the new Sloan-Kettering model were released or forced out. Some members of the health care community contend that Sloan-Kettering has been harmed as a medical institution because of Marks's policies and philosophy. "Marks is a kind of administrative Rambo," says Dr. Jerome DeCosse, a surgeon at New York Hospital and formerly chairman of surgery at Sloan-Kettering's Memorial Hospital. But DeCosse and all of Marks's detractors add quickly that in terms of operating funds — in terms of the all-important bottom line — Sloan-Kettering has never been healthier.

Haber, though, disagrees with Marks's approach.

Medical accomplishments grow out of holistic research. One of the things that I aimed for and that we accomplished at Massachusetts General was to be strong in all areas of cardiology. I tried my hardest not to tilt the cardiac unit solely in the direction of the interests of the chief, as some other hospitals do. My main goal as head of cardiology was to be sure that everything which is important to patient care was represented in the department, not only in someone competent to carry out patient care but also in someone skilled at bringing his or her enterprise to the forefront of research and the cutting edge of knowledge.

A bias toward a holistic approach may be at the heart of the way Haber organized his unit at Massachusetts General, but he also admits that some of his earliest impressions as a physician made it inconceivable that any cardiology department he led would be without an arrhythmia component.

Some of my bleakest memories of my internship in the late 1950s are of the times when we made rounds in the Critical Care Unit and we'd find people dead in bed from an arrhythmia, perhaps fifteen or twenty minutes after they'd last been seen fine and happy by the nurse. I was determined that we would someday know enough about what was happening to these patients so that we could prevent it.

Arrhythmias are such an important part of cardiology I couldn't conceive of having a broad and general cardiac service without a very major effort in arrhythmology in respect to both patient care and research. In inviting Jeremy Ruskin years ago to start the Arrhythmia Service I very much had in mind that we could not move ahead without that being a very important part of our department.

Haber's distinct management style is perfectly in character with the rich history of Massachusetts General, a hospital known for going against the grain in the way it practices medicine. Massachusetts General is the oldest voluntary nonprofit hospital in New England and the third oldest in the United States.

The first patient entered Massachusetts General in 1821; since then more than four million of the region's and nation's sick have been cared for there.

At its inception, Massachusetts General, which is currently spread out over twenty structures, was crammed entirely into the Bulfinch building, now a tourist attraction and research center that houses the offices of the Arrhythmia Service in its basement. The Bulfinch was named for its designer, Charles Bulfinch, Boston's first native-born architect and the man who designed the Massachusetts State House, located nearby. The Bulfinch is a massive structure made of white-hot Chelmsford granite, with a portico of eight huge Ionic columns; it is topped at its four corners by industrial-strength smokestacks. But beyond its imposing classical architecture, the Bulfinch signifies a great moment in medicine. There, on October 16, 1846, health care's boundaries were dramatically and permanently altered.

On that day at Massachusetts General, modern, painless surgery was launched. High up in the dome of the Bulfinch — in the amphitheater reached by climbing either of two winding cantilevered staircases with colonial lanterns hung on their walls — dozens of physicians and researchers watched from the auditorium as a white mask was placed over the mouth and nose of a patient about to undergo surgery to remove a tumor from the side of his jaw. Dr. William T. G. Morton, a local dentist of some renown, uncorked a series of pipes leading into the patient's mask and ether streamed into a patient's lungs and bloodstream. A moment later, Morton carefully examined the patient, closed the patient's eyes, and said quietly to the physician standing beside him, "Your patient is ready, sir."

Standing in the wide-open vistas of the dome, reliving that October day, it is hard not to imagine the spectators gasping quietly, leaning forward intently, and straining to get a glimpse of the unconscious patient. Dr. John Warren, Massachusetts General's first surgeon and a cofounder of the hospital, nodded to Morton, picked up his scalpel, and proceeded to cut the patient's jaw open. The spectators winced in pain — it was impossible for them to comprehend and accept the fact that the patient felt nothing and was numb to the sharp blade of the scalpel. Within an hour the operation was completed. Soon after, the patient was conscious, fully recovered from the effect of the ether, his surgery successful.

Warren turned to those in the gallery and bellowed: "Gentlemen, this is no humbug." The dome above him emphasized each of his words with a strident echo. Within a year of this landmark operation, ether was commonly used worldwide. Not long after, Dr. Oliver Wendell Holmes, who had watched the operation that day, coined the term anesthesia, combining *an* — absence of — with *aisthesis* — sensation. And because of that day in 1846, the Bulfinch amphitheater became known as the Ether Dome, a term that is still synonymous with turning points in medicine.

Since then physicians at Massachusetts General, inspired by the achievement in the Ether Dome, have continued to take on and obliterate medical obstacles. The list of innovations that were pioneered at Massachusetts General reads like a box score of research leapfrog played by each succeeding generation of physicians and clinicians. For example:

- In 1869, Dr. J. Collins Warren, a grandson of the John Warren who held court in the Ether Dome in 1846, introduced the techniques of sterile surgery to the United States.
- In 1886, Dr. Reginald Fitz identified appendicitis, an age-old disease. Fitz's research kicked off an era of successful appendectomies. More important, though, to perform appendectomies surgeons had to open the abdominal cavity, which until then had been strictly off limits to invasive medical treatments.
- In 1925, the first tumor clinic in a hospital was founded at Massachusetts General.
- In 1926, Dr. Joseph Aub discovered the cause and treatment of lead poisoning.
- In 1929, a team that included Drs. Oliver Cope and

Fuller Albright performed the first successful operation to cure hyperparathyroidism, a common endocrine-system disorder.

- In 1937, physicians at Massachusetts General, in conjunction with researchers at the Massachusetts Institute of Technology, used radioactive iodine in thyroid studies and launched the era of nuclear medicine.
- In 1962, Dr. Ronald A. Malt attached a severed human arm.
- In 1981, Massachusetts General researchers and those at MIT and the Shriners Burns Institute invented artificial skin.

No discipline, though, fared better than cardiology at Massachusetts General. The history of cardiology at the hospital is especially colorful, thanks especially to the antics and the medical genius of Dr. Paul Dudley White, who was more comfortable upending traditional clinical principles than resting in the safety of tried and true — too often meaning stagnant — health care concepts.

Paul Dudley White, known as P.D. to most of the people he came in contact with, was a five-foot-four, 120-pound whirlwind. White literally hauled cardiology into America box by box, when in 1914, as a young doctor returning from his studies in England, he brought with him one of the first electrocardiograph machines. He proudly installed this cumbersome tangle of electrodes and saline buckets — the electric impulse conductors into which the patient's limbs were dunked — in a small closet deep in the basement of Massachusetts General's Skin Hall. Immediately, White was teased mercilessly by his former medical school classmates and his older colleagues. Many years later, White would say, "The machine was viewed with suspicion and even subject to an unusually high amount of derogation by most of the doctors."

The contraption was also nearly completely ignored as a diagnostic tool by many of the practicing physicians at Massachusetts General. White, though, used it extensively on patients and then opened himself up for more ridicule a year later, when he somehow convinced the hospital leadership that he should be allowed to found a Cardiac Unit at the hospital, the first such department in the country. (The sales technique he used on Massachusetts General administrators was apparently incessant nagging until he wore down the opposition.)

P.D.'s colleagues regarded cardiology as a paltry, insignificant medical subspecialty. Indeed, cardiology was viewed with such disdain that Massachusetts General physicians saw it as nothing more than pure entertainment when White and his entourage descended on the wards like a flock of geese to visit patients. Dr. Edward Bland, who would succeed White as head of the Massachusetts General Cardiac Unit thirty-four years later and who was an admirer of White from the beginning, recalls that the attitude of the hospital's doctors toward these twice-weekly patient/doctor sessions was something far less than professional.

White and his cardiac group would make the rounds in our ward every Tuesday and Friday morning at ten-thirty. White bolted in first, moving faster than everybody around him — nobody could keep up with him — usually followed by a group of students, associates, and visitors. It was quite an event on the medical service — one that was never taken seriously and that led to plenty of pretty aggressive joking in its wake among the staff.

Interestingly, seventy years later electrophysiologists would be subject to the same disdain — this time, though, by cardiologists, practitioners themselves of a subdiscipline that was once outcast but that is now a part of the conservative mainstream of established medical thought.

White was not oblivious to the response that his activities evoked, but he was so confident about the clinical path he had chosen that he always knew he would be vindicated eventually. Indeed, as a classics and history major in college before settling on medicine, P.D. understood from historical and literary precedent that the best ideas are usually the ones allowed to germinate and develop out of favor or in disrepute. From Gutenberg to Mozart, White once told a friend, those with something important to offer were derided. The only thing that is important in medicine as well as life, he added, is long-term results, not the petty jealousies and reprobation one suffers along the way.

White's optimism was just the tonic cardiology needed to emerge as a foundation of modern medicine. He was an excellent spokesman for the fledgling subspecialty, and he nurtured it brilliantly. His unflagging optimism set the tone for the subtle and not so subtle alterations of medical thought that he promulgated with such flair and persistence — and that he backed with logic and evidence. Before long White's ideas could not be ignored by the health care community.

Perhaps P.D.'s most important contribution to medicine was the notion that heart disease is not a death notice, pure and simple. Most cardiologists of his period offered their patients the prospect of nothing more than an existence of semi-invalidism, in which they awaited their next heart attack as if they were marked for imminent death, and in which only an extremely sedentary existence could forestall the Black Angel for a limited time. White termed this attitude "poppycock" and did so often. He stressed to his patients that there are many different physical conditions — none is necessarily the "normal" one — and that, properly managed, heart disease and nonaverage cardiac function need not debilitate a patient.

To prove his point, P.D. recorded the pulse rates of ten runners just before the start of the Boston Marathon in 1917. A few had heart rates as high as 118 — clearly "abnormal" by most measures — while others had pulses beating at an extremely low 60. White reveled in these findings.

If a heart rate of over 100 had been a criterion for excluding participation in the race, we would have rejected the winner, who finished this long race easily and comfortably.

White followed this study with numerous others, dispelling many myths about heart disease. He played a key role in furthering the concept, for example, that the clogging of arteries by fatty deposits was not solely the result of aging but also of an inactive life-style and poor nutrition. Countering the advice of most of his colleagues in and out of cardiology, White emphasized, long before it became chic to do so, that exercise and good eating habits are important contributors to cardiac strength and health.

Despite the view of many skeptics and the absence of voluminous statistics to prove that physical exercise prolongs life or prevents or delays presenile atherosclerosis of coronary or cerebral arteries, there are clear physiologic reasons for its beneficial effect on the circulation in healthy individuals as well as in the majority of patients with chronic disease. Although a strong and supple heart muscle is the major factor in maintaining an optimal circulation in the human body, there are certain accessory pumping mechanisms that are rarely spoken of, let alone emphasized.

White felt that the most important "accessory pumping mechanism" is the musculature of the legs, particularly that of the thighs. When thigh muscles contract during activities that use the legs extensively — such as walking, swimming, bicycling, soccer, and basketball — the blood is pumped briskly upward from the feet through the leg veins toward the heart against gravity.

The standing, sitting, or recumbent position, which requires little, if any, use of the leg muscles, leads to a sluggish circulation or stasis of blood or of its watery content in the feet and ankles. On the other hand, active contractions of the legs can account for about one-third of the circulation, relieving the heart of some of its work load.

Another muscle that White singled out as essential to proper working of the heart and one that can benefit from extensive exercise is the diaphragm.

I am always more optimistic about a patient's future when I observe through the fluoroscope a free and full excursion of the diaphragm during respiration, bringing not only ample air into the lungs but, by negative pressure on the thorax, also aiding blood flow to the heart.

A sedentary program, P.D. pointed out, a high diaphragm pushed up by too much abdominal fat, or down by pulmonary emphysema due to smoking, significantly reduces full ventilation of the lungs and may impair the flow of blood back to the heart. In those cases where the movement of a patient's diaphragm seemed stilted, White often initiated a program of periodic deep breathing to ease the problem.

P.D. didn't merely tout the value of exercise, while living otherwise. He practiced what he preached. His bicycle was his most frequent form of transportation around Boston; his frugal diet — lunches of peanut butter on crackers and bouillon, breakfasts of toast with margarine — was his trademark.

Combined with his constant proselytizing for preventive medicine were boundless energy and an insatiable appetite for amassing more and more data about the heart. The stories about White as cardiac researcher and writer are legion; they sound suspiciously apocryphal but the facts dispel any disbelief. In 1928, for example, White and his wife of four years left Boston on a traveling fellowship through Europe. Somehow, in between sight-seeing and studying, White found time to write a 931-page book called *Heart Disease,* which quickly became the definitive work on the subject. Contrast that achievement with the response thirty years later when White tried to persuade two younger colleagues to coauthor a new edition of *Heart Disease.* The junior physicians begged off the project, taking refuge behind their heavy schedules. White looked at them with disbelief.

I get some of my best work done after ten or eleven o'clock at night. You get three or four hours of good work, and you'll be surprised how fine you feel when you get up at six o'clock. Then, after two or three years the book will be finished, and you'll scarcely have noticed the effort.

There are other stories about White, equally larger than life. One night after a long day at Massachusetts General, P.D. was seen by the General Director of the Hospital, Dr. Nathaniel Faxon, sneaking into the autopsy room. A few hours later, seeing the lights still on in the room, Faxon entered and witnessed an unforgettable scene. As he recalls it, it was either the portrait of a scientist driving himself beyond the normal call of research to a brink of remarkable achievements or a scientist literally drowning himself in rapidly rising pools of data.

There was Dr. White, sleeves rolled up, in hip boots, slopping around, exploring the heart of a dead elephant. I thought he was crazy. Or a genius. Or both. Above all, I do recall that he was completely happy.

White looked at Faxon, oblivious to the General Director's quizzical expression and his attempt to assess the sanity of the cardiologist. White shoved his hand farther into the tissue of the elephant's heart, boasting loudly, "Look, Nat, it's just like a human heart — but see its size. I can put my two fingers in the coronary artery."

Though it was perhaps not immediately apparent, there was a great deal of logic behind White's incursion into the elephant's heart. P.D. was curious about the dissimilarities between the huge, sluggishly beating heart of a large animal like the elephant and the tiny, jackhammer-paced heart of a small animal like the mouse. In the end, he was trying to delineate the role that size difference plays in the entire range of cardiac functions, findings that could be transposed into notions about the human heart.

White's search for the animal kingdom's cardiac secrets ultimately took him far beyond that autopsy room at Massachusetts General. In the 1950s, when White was already in his late sixties, he booked passage on numerous whaling vessels to pursue the perfect EKG recording of whales. Using electrodes shot out of rifles or transported by harpoons, P.D. took aim at the ocean mammal, hoping to track the rise and fall of its heart rate and cardiac rhythm as it bucked waves and glided through the waters. The larger whales eluded White, but he did succeed in obtaining some EKGs of smaller whales.

Nothing medically earthshattering grew out of P.D.'s experiments with animals — heart-to-heart comparisons and correlations based on cardiac size are exceedingly difficult, because that property of the heart pales next to genetic makeup, tissue strength, environmental conditions, and the adequacy of the circulatory system as a factor in determining the long-term health of a person's or animal's heart. But White's well-publicized chase of the whale, which captured the fancy and attention of the lay public, perfectly buttressed his lifework and his efforts to enshrine cardiology as one of the most vibrant and up-to-date branches of medicine.

Through it all, though, even as his celebrity grew, White was attentive to his patients and their needs. They were his and medicine's raison d'être, he stressed, and that must never be forgotten, lest hubris taint health care irrevocably. A colleague of P.D.'s notes that it was typical of a busy medical teacher to bustle into a patient's room, remove the chart from the corner of the bed and, back to the patient, discuss the case with hovering students. Not so White.

Paul White was just the opposite. He always spoke first to the patient, talked to him in an understanding manner, and after making friends with him and discussing the character of his problem, he would pick up the chart and ask questions of the interns, residents, and students, still facing the patient. In this way he showed that he considered the patient as an individual. He would literally go to any ends to help a patient or do what the patient asked of him.

In 1949, after a thirty-year tenure as chief of cardiology at Massachusetts General, P.D. relinquished the office to his long-time friend Edward Bland. White devoted the rest of his life to writing, preaching often about the virtues of preventive cardiac medicine, and caring for patients locally, nationally, and internationally. Indeed, by the 1950s White had become such an essential U.S. resource that when President Dwight Eisenhower suffered a heart attack in 1955, P.D. was summoned to treat him.

And through it all, White never lost his insatiable curiosity and thirst for commenting on the trends and foibles of modern life and how they affect long-term health. A letter he wrote to the *New England Journal of Medicine,* when he was 86 — just a year before he died — perfectly captures the sly, tongue-in-cheek sense of humor, depth of knowledge, and human concern that he never lost. It was called "The Tight Girdle Syndrome":

During the last year or two I have become acquainted with the tight-girdle syndrome, which has fascinated me. It arises from the attempts of a rather stout woman to contain herself within some bounds of shapeliness. It has three aspects that have brought it to my attention.

First of all, on a number of occasions I have been puzzled by finding a vigorous carotid pulse accompanied by a jugular pulse visible just about at the edge of the right clavicle. The rest of the examination of the patient has shown no physical abnormality of the heart or blood vessels to explain this unusual pulsation in the neck. But when on occasion I have asked the patient to loosen the girdle, this pulsation has disappeared, much to my satisfaction and relief and to that of the patient, too, who now breathes more easily and feels less choked up.

The second aspect of the syndrome is gastrointestinal, with a displacement upward of diaphragm, stomach and esophagus, causing symptoms that are often attributed to a hiatus or diaphragmatic hernia with or without heartburn and gaseous eructation and commonly called cardiospasm. Again loosening the girdle relieves some of the symptomatology.

And thirdly it is quite obvious on fluoroscopy to see that the diaphragm is pushed up, and the heart displaced upward to assume a horizontal position, with a decrease in the thoracic space for the function of the lungs and of the heart. Dyspnea can result, relieved again by loosening of the girdle.

The tight-girdle syndrome is doubtless a residual of the popularity of the wasp waist that was in style a couple of generations ago, pictured in many of the fashion magazines of the époque. Perhaps now that women have been liberated they may be able to be free of the feeling that they need tight girdles.

On August 12, 1974, White and his wife bicycled through the streets of Lexington and Concord and then ate at the Concord Inn. Early the next day, P.D. suffered a massive stroke. He died on October 31, leaving behind an era of medical achievements unparalleled by any other physician in history.

P.D. White is nothing less than *the* inspiration for the Cardiac Arrhythmia Service at Massachusetts General. Jeremy Ruskin says that White's influence pervades the entire Cardiology Unit at Massachusetts General.

The tradition of great clinical cardiology and the patient as the center of attention, the tradition of focusing research on clinically relevant questions and practical answers to heart disease is White's legacy. It permeates the environment at the Arrhythmia Service and is in large part responsible for the extraordinary depth and breadth of expertise in cardiology at Massachusetts General.

·7·

Basement Notes from the Bulfinch: The Case of Ma Bell's Highflier

I N 1983, when American Telephone & Telegraph was forced to let go of the Baby Bells, the local phone companies, much was written about how the breakup would affect consumers and businesses alike, but nothing was said about the real victims, the "long-termers" at AT&T, who suffered tremendous emotional pain and pressure as they stripped their company of the wealth and power that they had given their lifetimes to building. One of these victims was sixty-three-old Jeffrey W., a stocky, active man, who led a full life, jogging through the streets of his Southern New Jersey town one day and piloting single-engined planes from a small Reading, Pennsylvania, airport to Oshkosh, Wisconsin, the next. The courts' decision to carve AT&T into smaller pieces changed his life immeasurably.

I was in planning and marketing for Bell. I loved my job and never expected it to destroy my health. But all of a sudden, after Judge Greene announced that AT&T had a short time to divest itself of its regional subsidiaries, I was thrown into a work schedule that was impossible to keep up with. Six- to seven-day weeks of twelve- to fifteen-hour days for months at a time. I began to eat irregularly and on the run, if at all. I stopped exercising and flying. And I was under terrific pressure to meet unmeetable deadlines as I tore apart a corporate giant that I was proud of. All of us at AT&T were suffering together and it affected each of us differently.

There were both outwardly apparent and inwardly felt manifestations of the toll that the Bell breakup was exacting from Jeffrey W. His weight, which he had always struggled to keep within strict bounds, climbed inexorably. And he experienced daily bouts of fatigue and torpor. He paid no heed, though, and chalked it up as the temporary result of overwork.

But on a cold, dismally gray December afternoon, Jeffrey W. found out how permanent the damage from overwork was. While he was having a cavity filled at his dentist's office, sharp stabs of pain begin to radiate from the middle of his chest down into his diaphragm. They came with a vengeance, then subsided, but kept returning, each a little more forceful than the one before.

"I thought it was indigestion," Jeffrey W. recalls. "I didn't say anything about the pains to the dentist."

On his way home in his car, the abrupt jolts in his chest worsened and lasted for longer and longer periods. Soon, they were constant. Jeffrey W. decided that something was definitely amiss and he drove to his doctor's office. The receptionist told him that the doctor was fighting his way through an exceptionally busy schedule but that she would try to fit him in. She asked Jeffrey W. to take a seat in the waiting room.

He sat their patiently, telling himself in every way he could that he only had a bad attack of indigestion, that everything would be all right. But the chest pains refused to subside — indeed, they continued to worsen. After another few minutes, he had no choice but to admit it — something was clearly very wrong. Jeffrey W. struggled slowly to the receptionist's booth, looked into her eyes and said softly: "Look, I'm in bad shape, I've got to see the doctor right now."

The receptionist called the doctor over the intercom. He rushed out, took one look at Jeffrey W.'s ashen face, touched his heart with the stethoscope, and said abruptly, "Get an ambulance! He's got to get to the hospital quickly!"

On the way to the hospital, the emergency team monitored Jeffrey W.'s heart, watching the electrocardiograph readout for any signs that its performance was flagging. There were none, and there was no indication that he was suffering from a cardiac arrhythmia.

Jeffrey W. actually began to feel a bit better. The chest pains seemed to have eased off. He knew that he had suffered a heart attack, but it seemed too minor to kill him, so he wasn't concerned at all about that. Instead, one thought kept gnawing at him.: "I'm going to lose my pilot's license. They're going to take it away from me. Heavens, what am I going to do without it?"

He could not rid himself of this thought. With this calamity, he felt, the ability to enjoy the life he had chosen could be taken from him.

By the time he arrived at the hospital, the worst of Jeffrey W.'s heart attack seemed to be over. He was given drugs to keep his heart rhythm stable and was told he would have to remain in the Cardiac Care Unit for several days while a battery of cardiac tests was run. There was still no definite diagnosis or prognosis of his disease.

Jeffrey W. was feeling positively chipper, almost invincible. "I survived the big one and it wasn't that bad," he thought. He recalls looking around at the patients in his ward and growing sadder and sadder about their conditions. He kept telling himself, "These people are in dire shape. They've got big problems."

It was early in the morning, not much past dawn, of his second day at the hospital when something happened with such suddenness that he had absolutely no time to react. Two or three breathtaking blows assaulted his chest. It was like being hit by the combined rights at full tilt of Joe Frazier and Muhammed Ali. Then he was unconscious.

The emergency cardiologist was summoned while the hospital staff performed cardiopulmonary resuscitation and tried to keep him alive.

When the cardiologist arrived in the room, a few minutes later, an intern stopped him at the door. "Don't bother, he's gone."

"The hell he is," the cardiologist said and pushed the intern out of his way.

Standing over Jeffrey W., the cardiologist looked at the vital signs monitors and at the electrocardiogram. He said to the nurses, "Prep him for an angioplasty."

It was clear to the cardiologist that Jeffrey W. was suffering from a cardiac arrest due to a massive myocardial infarct. One of the major coronary arteries feeding his heart was blocked with atherosclerotic plaque, so that oxygenated blood was unable to reach the cardiac muscle. An angioplasty, commonly known as cardiac balloon therapy, involves threading a catheter with an inflatable balloonlike tip through the narrowed artery until it reaches the area of blockage. The balloon is then inflated, flattening the fatty plaque against the arterial wall, and reopening the vessel to allow restoration of blood flow through it.

The angioplasty was an immediate success. Once again Jeffrey W.'s vital signs returned to normal and he rested comfortably. But this reprieve was short-lived. Nothing that had happened up until that point prepared him for the events to come.

Jeffrey W.'s massive heart attack and cardiac arrest left in their wake a severely damaged heart. So much so that when he was brought back to the CCU after the angioplasty, his blood pressure began to drop again. He was put on a respirator, given sedatives to ease the discomfort, and monitored constantly.

I guess that was the most horrible thing I ever went through. I was going in and out of consciousness. Often I knew what was going on around me and I could hear people talking, but I was strapped down and so weak that I couldn't move to respond or join in. It was as if I was a spectator in a world in which I was the center of attention.

Gradually, Jeffrey W. became so languid and felt so completely separated from the flow of day-to-day living that he was willing to accept the end. He said to himself, "I've had a pretty good life. This isn't a bad way to go. Just let go."

His mind wandered to what he would miss about being alive and what he wouldn't regret leaving behind. Suddenly, a thought occurred to him: "Wait, I can't die yet. My daughter is getting married next September. This is the happiest time in her life. I can't pull this on her."

Whether it was a case of mind over matter or a simple miracle superseding medical expectations and know-how no one can say, but within minutes the physician on the CCU was in the waiting room telling Jeffrey W.'s wife: "We have absolutely no explanation for it, but his vital signs are improving."

Another reprieve for Jeffrey W., yet just the beginning of a new round of hard times. Even while life was returning to his body, Jeffrey W.'s heart was so debilitated that it could barely support him. What is worse, an arrhythmia — ventricular tachycardia — took up residence in his damaged, vulnerable cardiac muscle.

And with the arrival of the tachycardia, the sadly familiar and misapplied clinical strategy of prescribing numerous randomly chosen anti-arrhythmia drugs until one worked, practiced by cardiologists unfamiliar with the breakthroughs in electrophysiological techniques, was implemented. Initially, Jeffrey W. was given an experimental but promising anti-arrhythmia drug that seemed to reduce the severity of his tachycardia but did not suppress it completely. Still, his physicians hoped that over time it would control the arrhythmia. Prescribing large doses of the drug, they finally released Jeffrey W. from the hospital, five weeks after he was first admitted.

It was a snowy, blustery, depressing day in January 1984, when Jeffrey W. left the hospital. Though he finally had his freedom again, this was not exactly what he'd had in mind when on that bed in the CCU he made the decision to continue living. Now confined to a wheelchair, he felt like only half a man. His virility, his ability to fly and jog and travel freely, all of the joys that sustained him, were stripped away.

This was never more apparent than, literally, the moment he arrived home. As his wife, Dorothy, turned their station wagon into the driveway, it skidded, swerved, and then got stuck in the center of a snow bank half-way to the garage. Slipping in the snow and summoning all her strength, Dorothy lifted Jeffrey W. onto his wheelchair and pushed the uncooperative contraption through the snow into the house. Then she went back outside to clear the snow and move the car into the garage. Jeffrey W. recalls the sheer impotence of that moment with a shudder:

> That was the first time through my whole ordeal that it was really apparent that there wasn't a thing I could do to help my wife anymore. In fact, not only would she have to take over all the physical work that I did, but she would also now have the added burden of taking care of me. I went into the front room and had to look out for the first time in my life at my wife trying to shovel the car out and there wasn't a darn thing that I could do. At that point I really thought that life for me was going to consist of hobbling around the front room of my house, looking out the window in my pajamas.

Jeffrey W. was determined to overcome the effects of his heart attack and return to an active life — and he went at it with a vengeance that few cardiac patients are capable of. Almost immediately he started attending a cardiac rehabilitation center. Beyond all of his expectations, within a week — after three sessions — he was walking, slowly but comfortably, and lifting things again. Within six months, remarkably, he was jogging three miles a day at the respectable pace of four miles per hour. And initially, at least, it appeared that the drugs were keeping his arrhythmia in check.

By the summer of 1984, though, the first signs of new trouble emerged. During exercise, when his pulse rate was driven up, his heartbeat became increasingly irregular. The arrhythmia had returned. Jeffrey W. brought this to the attention of his doctors, who added a second drug to his regimen.

The new drug did little good. Physical exertion had again become a chore, and held few rewards. Each time he jogged, the irregular pounding of his heart combined with dizziness and lightheadedness to make it nearly impossible to continue. Finally, it got so bad that he was taken to the hospital by an ambulance in the middle of a jogging session.

At the hospital, his heart was monitored again for a few days. Not sure how to deal with recalcitrant arrhythmias, the physicians prescribed more drugs to the point that Jeffrey W. was taking nearly thirty pills a day, and yet the arrhythmia was still not fully controlled.

This fact was made clear when he went on a plane flight with a friend. Although he had lost his license, Jeffrey W. was still able to pilot a plane if he had a flier with him. Soon after landing at a local Pennsylvania airport, the two men began to push the plane into a hangar, when suddenly all strength drained from Jeffrey W.'s body. His arrhythmia had returned. Though he stayed conscious throughout this bout with arrhythmia, Jeffrey W. was barely alert.

An emergency team was summoned, but treating arrhythmias was entirely out of their league. All the rescue squad could do was put Jeffrey W. in the ambulance and monitor him closely during a forty-five minute trip to the regional hospital. The arrhythmia continued with a vengeance and only finally dissipated at the end of Jeffrey W.'s ride in the ambulance.

Jeffrey W. was devastated. Nearly a year after his first cardiac arrest he was still on the treadmill of disease, no closer to a cure than the moment he nearly died months earlier.

Jeffrey W.'s physicians in New Jersey gave up on the case. In their minds, they had simply run out of traditional pharmacological options. The case had run a long and painful course of mainstream solutions with no satisfactory resolution, and it was clear to Jeffrey W.'s cardiologist that less-conservative treatments were in order. After investigating the electrophysiology labs across the country, the cardiologist turned his patient over to Jeremy Ruskin.

Ruskin examined Jeffrey W. in early October, on a clear day when the trees in New England were at their peak of fall color.

When Jeffrey W. was settled on the patient table, a physician inserted an electrode catheter into his femoral vein and under the watchful eye of a fluoroscope guided it toward his heart. After the electrodes were positioned in the heart, a series of stimuli were delivered in an attempt to induce an arrhythmia. Within minutes, Jeffrey W.'s heart was in arrhythmia. Quickly, an electrical countershock was delivered to shut down the arrhythmia. A moment later, Jeffrey W.'s heartbeat had returned to normal.

Ruskin then made a clinical choice, which in hindsight he regrets, but which at the time seemed appropriate. He decided to attempt to treat Jeffrey W.'s arrhythmia with yet another drug, instead of recommending surgery to excise the region of the heart causing the tachycardia. In this case, though, through electrophysiological testing, Ruskin felt he could be reasonably certain that the pharmaceutical chosen was one that would work.

You have to remember the surgical procedures that are used to treat arrhythmias carry with them small, but definite risks of major complications. Every once in a while a patient doesn't get through an operation. So we have to consider pharmacological options first.

For the next two weeks, Jeffrey W. was treated with daily doses of Amiodarone, one of the more efficacious but toxic anti-arrhythmic drugs on the market, and monitored around the clock for any signs of arrhythmias or adverse reactions to the medication. Neither appeared. So Jeffrey W. was brought back into the electrophysiology lab and again through catheter electrodes an attempt was made to induce the arrhythmia. The Amiodarone worked. Despite stimulation of Jeffrey W.'s heart through the electrode catheters, no tachycardia occurred.

The next day Jeffrey W. was released from Massachusetts General. Two days later he and Dorothy went to California to visit their children. It was there that the toxic effects of the Amiodarone appeared. First, Jeffrey W. broke out in hives, the result of sensitivity to the sun caused by the drug.

Next, he began increasingly to experience severe shortness of breath, even when exerting himself only slightly.

Dorothy and Jeffrey W. cut their West Coast junket short, and he immediately went to see his New Jersey physicians, who put him through a battery of tests and X rays. His cardiologist delivered the latest bad news, frustration etched on every word. "Your lungs are being damaged by the Amiodarone. I'm taking you off it immediately."

By telephone, Jeremy Ruskin recommended that Jeffrey W. return to Boston for surgery.

It was April 1986, and Jeffrey W. was back on the patient table in the Massachusetts General electrophysiology lab. Once again, an anti-arrhythmia drug had failed — this time it had thwarted the tachycardia but proved dangerously toxic and compromised Jeffrey W.'s health in new, deadly ways.

The catheter electrodes were again slipped into Jeffrey W.'s body and positioned inside his heart. The strategy this time was to map the locations from which the arrhythmias arose in his heart by moving the electrodes through the right and left ventricles and analyzing the spread of electrical activity during the tachycardia. Because Jeffrey W. wasn't taking Amiodarone anymore, the arrhythmia was easy to start up. In fact, during the two-and-one-half-hour mapping procedure two separate and clearly defined electrical trouble spots were found in his heart.

One was in the front wall of the left ventricle, where the normal flow of electricity was hampered by a large aneurysm or dilatation of the scarred ventricle at the site of his previous heart attack. The other arrhythmia was in a site in the upper region of the interventricular septum, the muscular wall between the left and right ventricles.

With the mapping completed and the matrices of his arrhythmias pinpointed, Jeffrey W. rested in the CCU ward, awaiting the operation to cut off the electrical power to the arryhythmias, which would take place in two days. In Jeffrey W.'s case, open heart surgery, rather than a less invasive catheter ablation was required, because he had a quite advanced aneurysm and heart muscle damage that had to be removed.

Ruskin told Jeffrey W. that he was encouraged by the mapping procedure and felt that his prognosis was excellent, although he added that there was a 40 percent chance that he would require some form of medication for the arrhythmia after the operation; however, the drugs would be far more likely to be effective than they had been before the surgery.

On the day of his operation, Jeffrey W. was scared — mostly because he wasn't feeling frightened enough. "They gave me so many tranquilizers that I didn't feel tense at all, although I knew that I should be afraid to the end of my wits. That really frightened me."

After Jeffrey W. was wheeled in, Dr. Mortimer Buckley, chief of cardiac surgery at Massachusetts General, joined Ruskin in the operating room. When the patient was anesthetized, Buckley opened his chest and exposed the heart. Electrode probes were inserted and with electrical stimulation his arrhythmias were induced again. This was done simply to double check the previously conducted mapping of the heart and make sure that the two arrhythmia sites about to be operated on were, indeed, the correct locations for surgery and tissue removal.

Dr. Buckley then excised the aneurysm and the nearby scar

tissue, which was the cause of one of Jeffrey W.'s tachycardias. Next, Dr. Buckley inserted a cryoprobe, a surgical instrument capable of freezing tissue, into the upper region of Jeffrey W.'s interventricular septum. An ice-cold, minus-sixty-degrees centigrade numbing emission was delivered to the site, resulting in permanent cessation of electrical activity in that region. Finally, repeated attempts to induce an arryhthmia with electrical stimuli were unsuccessful. At the end of this three-hour operation, no arrhythmia could be found in Jeffrey W.'s heart.

One week after his surgery, Jeffrey W. was back in the Massachusetts General electrophysiology lab for his final test. An electrode catheter was inserted into his femoral vein and positioned inside the right ventricle and, once again, electrical stimuli were delivered to the heart. To the delight of everyone in the laboratory, no arrhythmia could be started. Jeffrey W. was told that he would be going home in a few days and that he would not have to take any antiarrhythmic medication.

Ruskin arrived in Jeffrey W.'s room not long after, his usually reserved demeanor left behind in the laboratory. He talked freely, beaming as he spoke. "I want you to understand one thing. Please don't forget it. When you leave here, you can, within reason, do all the things you did before your first heart attack. Don't be afraid to return to an active existence."

That was all the encouragement that the persevering Jeffrey W. needed to hear. He was already walking around, his heart free of pain. And before he left the hospital a few days later, Jeffrey W. was doing a couple of miles a day up and down the hospital corridor.

When Jeffrey W. and Dorothy returned home to New Jersey he felt renewed, freed from the disease and illness that had gripped him for nearly a year and not afraid any longer that he might die soon. For the first time he realized how fortunate he had been.

I really struggled for a year. And suddenly I felt so good and not sick anymore — that was the key. I was well again. So I cried because I felt so damn fortunate. That's when I said, "Why me?" Why have I been so fortunate, when there were so many times it could have gone the completely opposite way and I could've been dead.

I sat down and wrote a letter to Dr. Ruskin. I just tried to bare my chest. It was difficult to write a thank-you letter because I realized that treating patients with severe heart conditions is what he does for a living; this is what he's expected to do; it's what he gets paid for. But at the same time I realized that he and his associates have developed and acquired certain special skills and I happened to be the lucky person who was treated with these skills. I wanted him to understand that I was aware that he was just doing his job, but from my standpoint, "Thank God you burned the midnight oil to devise and acquire the skills to care for me the way you did."

A year later Jeffrey W. had had no recurrence of the heart disease and arrhythmias that had plagued him throughout the previous year. To him, it feels as if his execution was stayed. He lost a year of his life but regained his health.

As for his pilot's license, he is caught in the middle of a struggle that is raging at the Federal Aviation Administration. The removal of the embattled administrator who decided on medical matters has left a void in the agency yet to be filled. Jeffry W. is hopeful, though, that the impasse will be settled soon.

"If everything goes all right," Jeffrey W. says, "we'll be flying out to Oshkosh, Wisconsin, in a few months to an air show. I plan to follow the air shows next year."

Still, he's grown less concerned about his pilot's license. The very thing that made him determined to overcome cardiac disease has paled in significance to being given a fresh term in this world.

"As long as I keep breathing with a good quality of breath and life I can hardly complain."

·8·

Misplaced Generosity and Ignorance

UNLESS you enjoy discussing economics, don't spend too much time around doctors, for their stories of clinical triumphs frequently give way to conversations about fiscal responsibility, payers, payees, and the labyrinthian regulations of Medicare and the medical insurance companies. It's an unavoidable fact: being a physician these days requires that you be adept at identifying and skirting economic landmines.

There are many doctors in this country who practice nonaggressive, nonduplicitous medicine; for this their reward is to struggle with the whims of a disorganized and unpredictable money machine. Without relief they wrestle with an impoverished system supported by an odd triumvirate — the Medicare program and federal health care policy makers; third-party insurers like Blue Cross and Blue Shield and the thousands of private, for-profit insurance firms; and hospitals and other physicians who blatantly abuse the Medicare, Medicaid, and third-party payer system by overprescribing overpriced medical care.

Each of these players, in varying degrees, is responsible for a health care system that avoids formal bankruptcy only because the impact of the staggering amounts of money being passed around is distorted by mirrors that hide the truth.

The result of all this is that the patient is often penalized for being sick — and the physician with good intentions is handcuffed. Unavoidably, the kind of medical care that the patient receives is frequently decided by financial and not clinical yardsticks. Says Jeremy Ruskin, "The dollars and cents issue restricts the number of clinical alternatives that we can explore before choosing a final approach for a patient and occasionally limits the specific options available to some patients."

A perfect example of the intricate relationship between doctors and the cumbersome economic structure of health care was hammered home again when, minutes after Ruskin performed a procedure that stabilized the rhythm of a patient's heart, the capriciousness of fiscal reality intruded on the pleasure of the moment. Ruskin sat dejectedly in his office staring at a white sheet of paper in his hand. His voice edged with frustration, Ruskin pointed to the memo he held and said:

When you shovel away all of the bureaucratese on this paper, the message is simple. The federal government is arbitrarily cutting its Medicare payments for all arrhythmia procedures at Massachusetts General by fifty percent. There's no logic or rhyme or reason for a fifty percent across-the-board hacking of our reimbursement. It will close us down.

A typical arrhythmia procedure is, by any measure, a bargain. Take the case of Margaret W., described in chapter 5. The salaries of the physicians and technicians participating in the operation cost only $1200, and the price tag for using the full array of laboratory and electrophysiology equipment and the numerous catheters that monitored and defibrillated Margaret W.'s heart was an additional $1200 — in no sense an enormous sum when stacked up against common prices for health care today.

If we get cut down to six hundred dollars for equipment, supplies, and hospital charges per procedure, we're stripped to nothing. The catheters alone cost well over a hundred dollars each and we can run through as many as three during a procedure in the cath lab.

What's more, Ruskin adds, Massachusetts, in an effort to keep medical costs down, is one of only a few states that have legislated a stranglehold that places hard and fast restrictions on every health care dollar charged and the additional costs cannot be passed on to the patients.

In Massachusetts, all physicians are bound by Medicare and Blue Shield formulas. Whatever these insurers decide to pay is what we get and nothing more.

Of course the $1200 figure is purely the so-called professional fees for the electrophysiological procedure itself. Tally up the time an arrhythmia patient is in the hospital before and after the procedure, the daily tests, the around-the-clock staff support, and the numerous other diagnostic measures, as well as the frequent need for implantable devices like the automatic defibrillator, or sophisticated cardiac surgery, and the total cost of treating a complicated arrhythmia may balloon significantly.

Fortunately for Ruskin and his patients, the Medicare cutback never took place. But the mere existence of the memo from the federal government — and its implied threat that an across-the-board cut, perhaps of smaller dimensions, may soon be in the offing — was enough to send a chill through Ruskin as he contemplated the future and measured his ability to generate enough revenues to keep the Arrhythmia Service functioning.

To Ruskin and others administering arrhythmia centers around the country, the issue of how to ensure that these frequently fledgling and, by some standards, disposable units remain operating in today's medical economic climate is paramount and all-consuming. Working against these electrophysiologists is the bias toward high-tech, high-priced medicine and a reimbursement system that favors short-term, non–critically ill patients, as well as diagnostic and treatment approaches supported by the more traditional health care deliverers. Indeed, an examination into what Ruskin and his colleagues are battling lays bare the cancer in the very underpinnings of the health care system — in what motivates it and in what makes it tick — and clearly indicates that this cancer may kill the most innovative, inexpensive, and life-saving medical breakthroughs and strategies, like anti-arrhythmia care.

The question of how medical costs are paid for in this country and the numerous opinions, foolish and wise, on how they *should* be paid for are at the core of a well-publicized debate that seems to have no conclusion and that points up no viable solutions. Yet, there are undertones in this debate that contain the first hints of what went wrong in the economics of medicine initially and why. It also, perhaps, offers a glimpse of what can be done to rectify an abysmal situation. Some questions that need to be answered are:

- What political and fiscal compromises between Congress, the insurance industry, and prominent physicians set in motion the essentially out-of-control Medicare system — the sorry role model for other reimbursement programs? Though it could not be seen twenty years ago, at its birth the Medicare system was the big bang that irrevocably altered the structure of health care's fiscal house.
- Who decides which clinical procedures and professional services are reimbursable by Medicare and third-party payees?
- What are the criteria used for deeming a particular procedure reimbursable?
- How do the disparate members of the health care com-

munity fit into and, at times, encourage its topsy-turvy fiscal environment?

The ground rules that led to the misshapen economic state of health care were laid arbitrarily twenty-five years ago in a fit of misplaced generosity and ignorance.

When President Lyndon B. Johnson first introduced Medicare legislation, in 1964, it contained a reimbursement plan for hospitals and physicians similar to that used at the time by Blue Cross and Blue Shield and other third-party insurers. Under this plan, health care providers would be paid according to a strict formula worked out by the insurance companies, not by doctors and hospitals. Reimbursement would be based on insurance industry tables that measured payouts against premiums and ensure that when the bottom line was computed the insurers would be in the black and the federal government would not be choked by the Medicare system. However, truculent lobbying from the American Medical Association killed this bill at its birth.

It became clear by 1965 that Medicare would not become law unless the legislation contained provisions for reimbursing physicians and hospitals with fees that were, to use the parlance of health care lobbyists, "reasonable," "customary," and in line with those "prevailing" in the community. Effectively, the bill would pass only if the reimbursement formulas were structured to ensure that the cost of medical care for senior citizens would grow wildly and rapidly become a high-ticket budget item.

Lyndon Johnson was sure that the nation's taxpayers could afford both guns and butter. So, despite the fact that the Vietnam War was draining the federal coffers, when the President was informed that Medicare could cost an additional half-billion dollars a year in 1965 (and many more billions during succeeding years) if the reimbursement formula were to be changed, Johnson laughed off any concern about the country's long-term ability to pay. He shrugged his broad shoulders and scoffed at the suggestion that perhaps the future budgetary implications of the amended Medicare legislation should be considered further. According to Joseph Califano, his health care adviser, Johnson told his Capitol Hill Medicare lobbyists: "Five hundred million. Is that all? Do it. Move that damn bill out now, before we lose it."

Johnson's offhand, thoughtless reaction to the rising cost of Medicare, even before it became law, changed the nature of health care economics permanently. The Medicare legislation legitimized for the first time the concept of reimbursement plans based on "reasonable," "customary," and "prevailing" rates in the medical community. And in the process, the control of reimbursement formulas shifted from the insurers to the health care providers themselves. The gravy train was off and running.

And it hasn't slowed down yet. Consider this: by 1985, health care's slice of the gross national product pie was nearly $400 billion, up from less than $30 billion twenty years earlier. This means that as a nation we spent over $1 billion a day on our medical care needs. It also means that health care topped 10 percent of the gross national product, felt by many analysts to be the threshold that separates a well-oiled health care delivery system from a dangerously disorganized and declining one. It is estimated that by the year 2000 medicine's percentage of the GNP will rise still higher, to 15 percent. What is more, 72 percent of this $400 billion was not paid out by patients themselves — that is, those receiving the services — but was reimbursement to physicians and hospitals from Medicare, Medicaid, the Blues, and private insurers.

Because health care providers exert considerable influence on the reimbursement formulas, the system has enabled physicians and hospitals to raise their rates annually at a pace double that of inflation since 1965 and has also shielded most individuals who receive the medical care from directly feeling the pinch of exorbitant prices. Yet, the indirect costs of this out-of-whack health care payment system affect us significantly everywhere. Half-a-million American cars and trucks have to be sold each year before the auto manufacturers foot their health care bills. Three cents out of the cost of every Mc-Donald's hamburger goes to insurance premiums for employees. Three dollars out of the cost of each $60 tire you buy goes directly to the health care industry. And the nation's trillion-dollar-plus debt is riddled with uncounted billions paid out to the health care industry.

And precisely because the escalating price of health care has been largely a covert menace, it has led to some outrageous buying and charging activities by physicians and hospitals. For instance, have you heard the story of the sixty-seven-year-old woman who was given a pregnancy test before routine surgery recently? The unskeptical Medicare administration apparently did not understand the joke that the physician played on his patient. It reimbursed the doctor $500 for his efforts.

And did you know that more than one hundred hospitals in the United States have their own helicopters, at a cost of over $1 million each or, if they are leased, at yearly operating expenses that can approach $2 million? Equipment like choppers is paid for almost solely by the insurance firms and government health care funds — though not directly. To afford such luxuries the hospitals overcharge reimbursers on nearly every item and service they provide. A patient's ride in a helicopter to the hospital — be it an emergency or not — costs his insurance company $2000; every Tylenol pill the patient takes is billed at sixty-nine cents; and cotton balls are one dollar each, according to many of the nation's hospitals.

Not all hospitals — and physicians — are recipients of such largesse, though. Massachusetts General is a tertiary care center for its region, and as such its mandate is to take in all patients who require critical medical support, who are so ill that end-of-the-road efforts are all that can be done. But MGH is in a state that regulates to the bone health care expenditures within its borders. Hospital budgets and charges are frozen and extremely limited; a noble gesture toward curtailing medical costs but unfortunately an ill-conceived one. Budgetary restrictions are based on a formula that severely impairs how much can be done for a patient using Medicare or other third-party money before the hospital is forced to pay the patient's bills itself. Long-term care is penalized in favor of short-term outcomes. And because Massachusetts General is saddled with the most complex long-term-care cases, its financial situation is growing bleaker and bleaker, while hospitals treating patients with less complex illnesses continue to thrive.

Hospitals like Massachusetts General received a similar slap from the federal government's recent attempt to limit Medicare reimbursements to hospitals, the so-called Prospective Payment System (PPS) begun in 1984. Under the PPS a hospital receives a fixed Medicare payment that depends on the physician's diagnosis but disregards the duration of the patient's stay. Though this is a well-meaning attempt to redress the blank check that Lyndon Johnson gave to health care providers in order to move Medicare through Congress quickly, Vincent Cucciero, Vice-President for Program and Facilities Development at Massachusetts General, notes:

> Because we get the sicker cases, our CCU beds are taken up by eighty-one-year-olds who are in heart failure of one form or another. There is no other place to bring them because they need the care. But the younger patients, those less critical, are sent elsewhere. It's the younger patients, however, with short-term needs that we can make money from; the elder patients, unfortunately, because of the way the system is structured, are a drain on the hospital.
>
> I saw one study recently that said that 80 percent of the total resources in the care of the elderly are used up in the last six months of life. But the Medicare system does not reimburse with those statistics in mind. So this becomes both a policy and ethical question. If you want us to continue treating the aged who are critically ill, the formula used to determine payments for their treatments should not be based on a general schema that crosses all demographics; it should be based on their special case.

In sharp contrast to Massachusetts General's fiscal woes is the economic health of many nontertiary hospitals in nonregulated states that continue to feast on Medicare, even with the introduction of the PPS cost-cutting measures — indeed, in some cases, ironically, *because* of the introduction of the PPS. This is because when the federal government set up the Prospective Payment System, in order to fend off lobbying from hospitals, it gave the health care community a tempting carrot: for the first time, it allowed hospitals to make a profit on Medicare — without having to be circumspect about it — by completing patient treatment for a particular diagnosis more quickly and under budget. For instance, Medicare will pay a hospital close to $5,000 for keeping a patient diagnosed as having uncomplicated heart failure in its cardiac care unit; this assumes an average stay of 6.8 days in the hospital. Now, suppose the patient's stay is cut to four days. Medicare will still pay $5,000 and the hospital pockets the $2,000 dollars it earned for releasing the patient nearly three days early; in addition, the hospital frees up a bed for the next Medicare patient.

It is no wonder, then, that in a recent survey of 236 hospitals, Richard Kusserow, the inspector general of the Department of Health and Human Services, found blatant examples of Medicare surpluses growing directly out of the PPS program. For instance, a 1,008-bed facility in Ohio made $30.3 million on $98.7 million of Medicare revenue. Worse yet, a 651-bed hospital in Missouri made $25 million on Medicare revenues of $58 million, a whopping profit margin of 43 percent.

Not blessed with the free lunch with which these other hospitals are endowed, Massachusetts General faces the reality of running a string of operating deficits for the first time in decades. To avoid this, MGH has had to come up with intriguing methods of raising money. For one, the hospital has entered into joint ventures with the private sector. As an example, Massachusetts General owns one-third of New England Health Resources, a high-technology home care company, and it is involved in a series of real estate ventures. But these for-profit activities are not considered a panacea.

"The reality is that the size of these joint ventures is minuscule when you look at the entire operating budget problem that the hospital is up against," says Vincent Cucciero. "The total Massachusetts General system of care is a half-a-billion dollars a year, and any of these joint ventures at most, if we're lucky, will spin off only two to three million dollars."

Another way that Massachusetts General is attempting to relieve its financial headaches is by good, old-fashioned cost cutting, something that some nontertiary care hospitals in unregulated states have not had to consider seriously. For instance, MGH now performs 200 kinds of operations on an outpatient basis. These procedures, on average, cost 75 percent less than they would if they were done during a two-day stay in the hospital.

Finally, Massachusetts General is using a more tried and true way to solve some of its problems: it is attempting to persuade state regulators to allow it to bring in some high-ticket, high-tech diagnostic and treatment tools that attract large numbers of patients for quick fixes and that carry very desirable reimbursements from insurers, even in Massachusetts.

Expensive high technology has always been a particularly attractive way to increase revenues for most hospitals and they've gone after it with an ardor bordering on the absurd. In a highly publicized incident in New York City three years ago, Sloan-Kettering requested the right from state regulators to buy a Magnetic Resonance (MR) scanner, which is used to detect tumors, head and neck injuries, and abscesses. MR scanners cost close to $1.5 million and are expensive to maintain.

The regulators denied the hospital its machine for a very logical reason: New York Hospital, across the street, had one already. Strong-armed pressure from Sloan-Kettering's politically powerful trustees followed, and within two weeks the regulators acceded to the hospital's wishes. Today, Sloan-Kettering's MR device is used on nearly two dozen patients a day at a cost of over $1000 per scan, reimbursable from third-party insurance companies and Medicare. By combining income from the MR machine with the MR's tax breaks from depreciation, Sloan-Kettering stands to profit handsomely from this particular excursion into high-technology.

And all of this in the face of some damaging information that has come to light about the MR device. Recently an expert government panel reported that "while MR is an extraordinary addition to our diagnostic armamentarium, it only has certain value in finding and identifying particular brain tumors." The panel then added that CAT scans, which cost $200 per patient, perform as well as MR for some patients and applications. Real and potential overuse of MR, the group noted, is cause for concern as doctors try aggressively to find new uses for the imaging technique. As one family practitioner said: "Some neurology clinics have become MR profit centers. You send them a patient with a headache, and they run up several thousand dollars of MR scans."

Massachusetts General had a similar experience with high-tech medicine a couple of years ago. One of the hospital's urologists told MGH administrators that there was a new device in Germany that could treat kidney stones without surgery, the lithotriptor. The administrators performed a careful cost/benefit analysis on the lithotriptor, comparing what the normal procedure for kidney stone removal was and how many hospital resources were used for it against what the new technology would cost and its effect. The cost/benefit workup showed that with the lithotriptor, hospital costs could be cut literally in half and, importantly for Massachusetts General, the number of cases that could be treated each year would rise from 100 to 1200; revenues from kidney stone treatments would be significantly enhanced. Fortunately for the hospital, state regulators bought its arguments for the lithotriptor and approved the device's treatment for reimbursement by third-party medical insurance carriers. As Vincent Cucciero recalls:

> It was clear that the lithotriptor's kidney stone removal technique made sense for full third-party and Medicare reimbursement, because there are only so many kidney stones in the world, you just don't go out and invent them.

The regulators know that on a global level Massachusetts General would be bringing in cases that would normally be treated at twice the expense at another community hospital. So there was a definite universal cost savings in our purchasing a lithotriptor.

ECMO, though, is, indeed, another story. In its zeal to augment revenues through gold-plated high technology, Massachusetts General is trying to convince state regulators that it should be allowed to purchase an ECMO (Extra-Corporeal Membrane Oxygenation) machine. ECMO is an artificial, out-of-body lung, akin to the heart/lung machines used during major operations such as coronary bypasses; it's an extremely questionable technique for curing the deadly, congenital lung problems suffered by severely premature babies.

ECMO is an example of one of the most controversial forms of high-tech medicine. And unlike the lithotriptor, with its definite constituency of patients with kidney stones, ECMO has an indefinite patient base. Infants are chosen by neonatologists to participate in ECMO treatments despite the fact that the technique has not proven its value and indeed has been shown frequently to be harmful. Millions of dollars in reimbursements await the physicians and hospitals that have ECMO at their disposal. Unfortunately, in this country's upside-down health care system, where quick-fix high technology is a revenue provider always and an efficacious form of health care only sometimes, ECMO has become the latest get-rich-quick scheme. But one only has to go as far as the nearest premature baby to be treated with ECMO to see how debilitating ECMO can be.

Take Lynda, a twenty-four-ounce premature baby, who was treated with ECMO after her birth a year ago. Her lungs were severely undeveloped and she was dependent on a respirator for breathing from her initial inhalation. As the hours wore on during her first day, Lynda's condition deteriorated. Her blood pressure decreased rapidly and such serious lung problems as persistent air leaks developed. Her chances of survival dropped literally with every breath that the respirator took for her. So after four days of distress, Lynda was put on ECMO.

But in order for her blood to flow unimpeded through ECMO, it had to be thinned, so it wouldn't clot and subsequently clog the artificial lung system. A chain reaction of clinical problems ensued. Lynda's unnaturally rarefied blood wreaked havoc with her immature circulatory system, which led to a series of massive brain hemorrhages. Now, one year later, Lynda is mentally damaged beyond repair. Because of cases like Lynda's, infants are no longer given ECMO if they show signs of intracranial bleeding. But this complication is not always easy to determine.

"Quite simply ECMO is a massively invasive procedure and we're trying to do it on some of the smallest human beings, who can't abide very much tinkering," says Peter Dillon, a senior surgery resident at Columbia-Presbyterian Hospital in New York City, who worked with ECMO through last year at the University of Michigan in Ann Arbor, where it was developed.

"When we talk to parents about using ECMO on their very preterm children," adds Dietrich W. Roloff, director of neonatology at Ann Arbor, "we tell them two things: 'One, ECMO may kill the baby; two, ECMO may help the baby to survive. You may be equally sorry in either case.' "

ECMO points up the most severe failings of this country's health care system. If hospitals and physicians are rewarded financially for embracing expensive new technologies that have not proven their clinical value, what follows is nothing short of an ultimate system-wide disaster.

For a medical technology or a clinical procedure to succeed these days, it must be reimbursable by Medicare.

"If Medicare doesn't cover it, hospitals don't buy it, physicians don't prescribe it, and patients don't get it," says Wayne Roe, an economist at the health care consulting firm, Lewin/ICF, in Washington.

The decision whether a new medical technology should be reimbursed by Medicare and thus be given the ticket to legitimacy and widespread use, rests for all intents and purposes with the Office of Health Technology Assessment (OHTA). To get a treatment, procedure, or technology covered by federal reimbursers, hospitals, physicians, and equipment manufacturers first send a petition to the federal Health Care Financing Administration (HCFA), which informs OHTA that an assessment should be made.

OHTA then begins an exhaustive investigation of the technology under consideration, taking input from a panel of physicians, clinical speciality groups, the National Library of Medicine, and any outside interested parties. Finally, a recommendation is made whether to reimburse or not, based on a consensus of opinions. While HCFA is not bound by the OHTA recommendation, there are few instances in which it has not rubber-stamped it without further consideration.

OHTA makes decisions about coverage; it does not evaluate the price of reimbursement. As Dr. Enriqué Carter, director of OHTA puts it: "Coverage is a decision about what you pay for; reimbursement is how you pay for it. We do not make decisions based on cost. We make decisions based on whether there is evidence that these technologies are reasonable and necessary for medical care. That's what the Medicare statute says that the decision is to be based on."

Unfortunately, the OHTA mandate is indicative of the woeful state of the nation's health care system. Because it ignores budgetary constraints, while making crucial recommendations about new medical technologies, it provides yet another example of how federal health care dollars are allotted with little regard for their ultimate toll on the fiscal house of cards. What's more, recommendations made by OHTA are heavily biased by the input of physicians, who in general support increased reimbursement for new technologies.

It would be difficult for OHTA to go about its business any other way. The agency is severely handicapped by an extremely low budget that precludes independent investigations of new technologies. With only $700,000 to spend in 1985 and $100,000 less to spend in 1986, it has had no choice but to rely on the medical community for advice.

For truly unbiased analyses of medical technologies to be made, it is estimated by the National Academy of Science that the federal government would have to allocate closer to $300 million annually.

"These funds would constitute much less than 1 percent of the country's annual medical bill," says Valerie Mike, clinical professor of biostatistics in public health at Cornell University Medical College in New York City. "The savings from eliminating useless or harmful procedures would far surpass this relatively minor investment."

Beyond the question of whether a particular technology is efficacious or not is the overriding one of whether we can absorb the cost — even if the outcome of using a medical advance is positive. At a time when we attempt to set harsh limits on the less expensive fruits of medical know-how, such as reimbursement for the time a physician spends listening and talking to patients, how can we justify a system that feels it need not even consider the *cost* of new technologies before recommending them for Medicare coverage?

"It's disgraceful that we're not willing to pay for the more fundamental medical accomplishments and are only willing to pay for big-ticket items," says Albert Jonsen, a professor of bioethics at the University of California, San Francisco. "There are a lot people dying in our health care system, and they're dying because they are not getting adequate care. They aren't dying because they've been refused the use of some latest piece of high technology."

Jonsen's point is illustrated graphically by the fact that one liver transplant, which costs about $150,000, could finance 30,000 office visits and treatments at an inner city clinic.

Comments like Jonsen's are the ravings of Luddites to much of the medical community. Still, there are those like OHTA director Carter, who is watching the inexorable march of medical costs from the inside, calling for a public debate on this matter — and quickly — before the health care system is paralyzed by its failure to properly define goals and priorities in line with how much money is available to pay for these goals and priorities.

There is a technological imperative that compels us to pursue new innovations in medical technology. There is also the tyranny of technology. More technology does not always equal better quality. Less is also not necessarily better or worse. Overall, we have to investigate the appropriate uses of medical advances before we implement them, and we have to examine our lack of willingness to unload ourselves of ineffective technologies. We are currently doing neither.

We must make some explicit societal decisions about what we aspire to in terms of quality of life and and quality of health care, and what we are willing to pay for them.

In the meantime, while this societal debate is on long-term hold, the health care system will continue to repeat its recent record of federal government indebtedness and inflated physician and hospital prices. And hospitals like Massachusetts General will attempt to shift gears as the rules of the game are altered, so that their programs can survive.

Says MGH administrator Cucciero: "We're in an Alice-in-Wonderland environment. Everything around us is changing so fast that one minute we're playing croquet and the next we're playing something entirely different. But the outcome is always the same. It's arbitrarily decided whether we win or lose, no matter how well we play the game."

Perhaps the most frightening aspect of the health care dilemma in this country, from a fiscal point of view, is that it is leading to renewed calls for national health insurance by many within and without the medical community. In some countries this would be a cause for celebration. In the United States, with its track record of give-backs and excessive reimbursements to health care providers every time it tries to provide free medical care, national health insurance would probably tear the economy to shreds.

Considering what health care costs already, it is incredible to listen to one administrator in a major New York City hospital describe his vision of the future:

> The fact that the Reagan Administration has proposed a catastrophic care policy for acute cases indicates that national health insurance is once more not a dirty phrase. Here's a conservative administration, preaching constantly that the government has no role in our lives, pushing a catastrophic acute care policy. That's very refreshing.
>
> Look, you have two choices: either go whole hog and pay for everybody's medical care, whether it be high-tech care or basic procedures, or let a large group of our population go without. I have a feeling we'll choose the former.
>
> One of the wise old men at this hospital told me recently that back in the early nineteen-sixties, hospitals didn't know where their next dollar was going to come from. And Medicare came along and saved the day. Well, we're having trouble now trying to figure out where the next dollar is going to come from to pay for all the new and old programs we want to fund — and things are only going to get worse. But when the attention gets firmly focused on this problem, I wouldn't be a bit surprised if we find the answer in more government-financed health insurance.

A scary thought, indeed. Enriqué Carter, at OHTA, adds, "We better change the direction of this debate quickly. You should never have some doctors, scientists, and bureaucrats sitting in a corner drafting society's future by themselves. We can't let the philosopher kings continue to set the health care direction for our society."

But can we let the public set health care policy? The Administrative Conference of the United States, an independent

Federal advisory panel, believes that we must. Recently, this group called for Medicare officials to publish a list of the criteria used for making decisions on reimbursement of new clinical technologies, and it added that the public should be given a channel through which it could comment on such national health care policy decisions.

It's unlikely that the federal government or Medicare officials will implement this recommendation of the Administrative Conference even though, at first blush, it appears to be a worthwhile notion. However, many health care insiders reject it outright. They contend strongly that if the public were allowed to make decisions about which clinical procedures should be paid for by government dollars, the result would certainly not be better — and perhaps it would be worse — than the situation that exists today.

As one leading cardiologist says: "The public wants everything at whatever cost when it comes to medical care — and it wants everything yesterday. If you think doctors are bad — and a lot of them are — turn this thing over to the public and you ain't seen nothing. Some of the implications in terms of where the public could lead us to fiscally if it decided on medical reimbursement are horrifying."

·9·

Cocaine and Arrhythmias: The Celtic Connection

THERE is a patient who nearly died from an arrhythmia whose case is more distressing than most, precisely because in this instance sudden cardiac arrest should never have happened. It was a pointless and confusing episode, marked by unexpected twists and serious questions about teenage drug abuse and abuse of power by adults. Setting the mysterious tone for this case was the physiology of the patient himself. As the physician on call in the hospital described it:

John T., to put it plainly, is an anomaly, at first glance anyway. For one, he's a teenager; most males who suffer sudden death by arrhythmia are thirty years old or older. For another, he's in good shape — an athlete — with no history of heart disease in his family. And finally, by the time we got to work on him, at least at cursory inspection, the arrhythmia had gone away completely — we simply couldn't detect it.

Two years ago, on an April night just before eleven o'clock, John T., a fifteen-year-old, strapping, good-looking boy with dark, strong features went into cardiac arrest. When he was rushed into the hospital he was unconscious, his heart having just recovered from a severe arrhythmic episode. Though it seemed an unlikely diagnosis, the first conclusion drawn by the physicians on duty was that the boy was suffering from cardiac disease that had not been detected previously.

But this diagnosis would prove to be faulty. Indeed, as John T. left the hospital a few weeks later, to everybody's surprise he walked out with a perfectly healthy heart. Unfortunately, he was impaired in other ways. Because the youth had been in ventricular fibrillation for a matter of minutes before his heart was successfully defibrillated by emergency medical technicians, he suffered brain damage from which he will never recover.

During the days that followed John T.'s admission into the hospital, a team of neurologists, cardiologists, and psychologists worked diligently to piece his story together. The police, the emergency medical squad who brought him in, numerous physicians, and John T.'s friends and family were all interviewed. Gradually, the mystery unraveled; the puzzle took shape.

In discussing the solution to the puzzle, John T.'s physician displayed unmistakable grief and anger.

John T. is a sick teenager who, by all odds, should not be suffering. No chronic arrhythmic condition exists in this patient. It was drugs that caused John. T.'s cardiac arrest from ventricular fibrillation and the subsequent brain damage; it was drugs and a moment of mental instability that, in this instance, was as damaging as the drugs.

The evening that would change the course of John T.'s life started uneventfully enough at the basketball court in the local schoolyard. The teenager and three of his friends, all of them top-of-the-class high school students with no police record and nothing but As and Bs on their report cards, went to the schoolyard to toss a few hoops before meeting their girlfriends downtown.

One of the boys smoked marijuana infrequently, not even enough so that it could be said he got high "socially." But tonight, with a lush springtime breeze seeming to wrap him in a soft, warm, invulnerable cocoon, he felt like getting stoned. He pulled a joint out of his pocket, lit it up, and passed it around.

John T. had never tried marijuana before, apparently more out of a fear of being caught and taken to task by his parents, prototypical pillars of the community, than of any real notion that marijuana was necessarily evil. This time, though he was goaded by no overt peer pressure from his friends, when the joint reached him John T. felt "courageous" enough to experiment in the safety of a schoolyard he knew singularly well. On a whim, he decided to try the pot.

Unfortunately, the basketball court was not as isolated and protected from view as he thought. As soon as John T. toked on the joint and inhaled it deeply, two school security guards emerged out of the shadows beyond the court's fence. The four teenagers were startled. John T. hurriedly dropped the joint and stepped on it. The security guards walked slowly toward the boys, menacing grins on their faces. The teenagers were cemented to where they stood, frozen in anticipation of trouble that couldn't be righted easily. Playfully, the security guards began to frisk the youths.

"Who's got the pot? Don't hold out on us."

None of the boys spoke. As the security guard frisking John T. reached his ankles, he looked toward the ground and saw the joint crushed at the youth's feet. The guard picked it up, examining it as he stood up. He said without emotion, "This boy was holding."

For John T., the next few moments were a blur. He remembers nothing except thinking about what his parents' reactions would be. How could he explain the complicated series of internal decision making that led him to his first innocent experimentation with a drug commonly used by teenagers, but anathema to his folks? His heart began to race out of control at the thought of this confrontation with his parents. Sweat poured from his skin. He was paralyzed in place and the danger didn't dissipate; instead it grew more menacing.

The security guards looked at each other. The one holding the joint, standing next to John T., laughed loudly.

"I think we ought to teach these boys a lesson."

John T. heard the click of handcuffs opening. His chest hurt. Sharp, wounding pains dipped from his heart through his arms and legs. And as the handcuffs closed on John T.'s wrists, he fell to the ground unconscious. He had suffered sudden cardiac arrest due to ventricular fibrillation.

The security guards tried to revive him but to no avail. One of his friends ran to the phone and called the ambulance. When the emergency medical team arrived, John T.'s heart was still fibrillating chaotically. Finally, moments later, it was defibrillated, and he was rushed to the hospital as he revived slowly.

John T. was released from the hospital two weeks later. He has brain damage due to a lack of oxygen to his brain during his fairly lengthy arrhythmic episode. His cerebral function will be hampered to some degree. Comprehension and response will be impaired, although how measurably is as yet uncertain. As for his heart, it is structurally normal, with no apparent heart disease and no detectable electrical abnormalities.

John T.'s case is an eye-opening affair that teaches numerous lessons about the unbreakable connections between drugs, heightened emotions, and arrhythmias.

There are a variety of possible reasons why drugs — especially cocaine and crack, less commonly marijuana — cause fatal arrhythmias.

For one, these drugs are stimulants. In addition to inducing euphoria, they sometimes cause significant increases in heart rate, blood pressure, body temperature, and metabolism. These factors — especially when they are present in dangerously high amounts, whether exclusively or in combination with other risk elements — can lead to arrhythmias.

More important, each of these drugs is capable of constricting the coronary arteries, the circulatory conduits that supply the heart muscle with blood and sustenance. This local and temporary cardiac blood deficiency, known medically as ischemia, produces profound electrical changes in the region fed by the constricted coronary artery and may lead to potentially fatal arrhythmias.

The final reason that drugs can unbalance the heart rate is that they interact and impair the user's nervous system on a physiological and emotional level. The brain — in particular the autonomic nervous system — exerts profound effects on the mechanical and electrical function of the heart. Because of this, drugs like cocaine and crack may dramatically affect the nature and quality of electrical traffic that reaches the heart and, consequently, cause a variety of adverse cardiac effects, including arrhythmias. Add emotional distress to the mood-altering capability of these drugs and the result is apparently a recipe for sudden death.

Indeed, this recipe is exactly what John T.'s body cooked up: the marijuana heightened his nagging fear of being seen as the good boy gone bad — of disappointing his parents by destroying the portrait he had carefully drawn of himself as an arrow that never strayed. And when the worst possible scenario for that night on the basketball court became reality — when the security guards discovered him on the wrong side of the good/bad spectrum and clasped the handcuffs onto his wrists — his nervous system, attacked by drugs and emotional distortion, began delivering chaotic electrical signals to his heart. A paralyzing arrhythmia ensued in a heart that was apparently normal in every way.

John T. is one of the thousands of anonymous young people who contract arrhythmias from drug use each year. Some die, some survive — many are harmed irrevocably.

One twenty-two-year-old who died in 1986 of cardiac arrest caused by a cocaine-induced arrhythmia was not anonymous in the least; in fact, he was front-page news and a shocking intimation for many young people of the uncompromising nature of mortality.

On June 17, Len Bias was standing proudly on a podium in New York City, a green Boston Celtics hat tilted on his head, his six-foot-eight-inch frame shyly and awkwardly posed for hundreds of clicking cameras. For the classy University of Maryland small forward with so much finesse, this was a moment to savor. His talent, his savvy, his dominating temperament on the court, his taut muscles and unswerving work ethic had enabled him to realize the dream of his life — to become a Boston Celtic, a member of the most successful professional basketball team in history. K. C. Jones, Bias's "coach for a day," described the twenty-two-year-old's aspirations simply: "Lenny had fallen in love with the idea of being a Celtic."

On the podium, Bias echoed this thought. He said quietly, "It feels good to be a Celtic."

And with that he walked off the stage and out of the hall, where the National Basketball Association draft was continuing. As he left, nobody could have imagined that this would be the last time we would see Lenny Bias alive. But that was the way it would happen. In a matter of hours, exultation was tranformed into sorrow. Less than two days later, Larry Bird, the soul of the Celtics, would say of Len Bias's sudden death, "It's the cruelest thing I've ever heard."

One man who certainly never expected his life to cross paths with Len Bias was Dr. Steven Geevas, the young emergency staff physician at Leland Memorial Hospital in Baltimore, a mere two-year veteran of the medical trenches. Geevas recalls reading about Bias, something of a local hero in Maryland, in the newspapers just before going to work about six in the morning on June 19. Accounts were given of how Bias took Boston by storm in a round of interviews not long after the New York City draft, of how everywhere he went in that basketball-mad town he was hailed as the next John Havlicek, a graceful, aggressive forward of an earlier Celtic era.

When Geevas arrived at the Emergency Room, it was unusually quiet. None of his colleagues — physicians or nurses — was around. But he dismissed this as a good sign that it was a slow day with few cases of any significance; he never suspected that anything was awry.

I changed into my hospital gear slowly and was reaching for a cup of coffee when one of the nurses ran out, panic written all over her face, and grabbed me. "Come into the arrest room immediately," she screamed. We ran into the room and when I walked in my heart started pounding. I knew immediately who this was. This huge black man was stretched out on the table — I had never seen a man that big sprawled out. He was unmistakably larger than life, if I may say so. But he was so near death.

It was at least an hour since Bias's cardiac arrest had occurred. When the emergency medical team had arrived to treat him at his University of Maryland dormitory thirty minutes earlier his heart was in ventricular fibrillation. The paramedics successfully defibrillated Bias before he was brought to the hospital. But although the chaotic beat had been stymied, in its place was no cardiac function at all. He was completely unresponsive, without respiration or pulse. As Geevas approached Bias, he was in what is known as asystole, total cardiac standstill.

Hurriedly, Geevas applied advanced cardiopulmonary resuscitation techniques. But the only response he was able to pry out of the young patient was yet another round of ventricular fibrillation. Quickly, Geevas injected Bias's heart with lidocaine, an anti-arrhythmic drug that usually works well in emergency situations, hoping to defibrillate him and, this time, restore a normal pulse. The effort failed. Bias's heart was defibrillated but once again went into asystole.

That was it. He remained that way throughout. I treated him for two hours but got no additional response at all. I gave it my best try and refused to give in, mainly because of his age. Young hearts don't die very easily, but his was dead from the moment he collapsed in his dorm room. I never really saw him alive.

In hindsight, Geevas admits that if he knew all the facts of the case he would perhaps not have treated Bias with lidocaine when his heart was fibrillating, because it is not a particularly effective approach for cocaine-induced arrhythmias. But when Geevas treated Bias there was no suspicion that this was a drug-related incident. Bias's roommates at the dorm took pains to hide any evidence of drug use before calling the emergency medical team, a time-consuming sideshow that stole from Bias his first precious moments after cardiac arrest, the few minutes a patient has to be resuscitated and live without neurological damage. Geevas explains:

> If you suspect that it's cocaine, then don't use lidocaine, treat with Inderal — that's the correct protocol. But you have to have an awfully good knowledge of what's going on to prescribe the right drug in this situation. The margin of error is exceedingly small and one has to act quickly. So we have to understand the situation very well. In this case, we had no facts and no suspicion of cocaine from any of the authorities on the case. But even if we did, he was in such full arrest and it was so long before the emergency medical team was even called that I do not believe in the least that we could have changed his course had we used Inderal.

When Geevas pronounced Bias dead, the Len Bias story was a confusing mishmash of rumors and hints. By that evening, the truth was emerging — and the story shocked the nation. Bias, the All-American success story, who transported himself from the concrete pallor of the playgrounds to the high glamor of the Celtics, had indeed snorted cocaine right before he died. When the klieg lights were brightest, he melted in the heat.

Initially, it was thought that Bias was a first-time user of the drug, but subsequent investigations indicated that he had depended on cocaine many nights and days of his short life. But what was different about his use of the drug on June 19 was that the pressure and anxiety — both positive and negative — had wound him tight and made him unnaturally high. Consider what had occurred to him in just a matter of days:

He went from being just another college basketball player to becoming the second-round draft choice in the nation, the pick of the Celtics. His best friend, Brian Waller, described how the mere thought of this achievement transformed Bias's usually even-tempered personality.

"He was pumped up, way too much so. He was unbelievably excited and nervous about going to New York and then Boston."

He also went from being a lower-middle-class youth to a man with a sure multimillion-dollar yearly income from his still-to-be-negotiated Celtics contract and endorsement packages, such as the one he signed with Reebok on June 18 just before returning to Maryland that, according to his agent, provided Bias with financial security for life.

In Bias's case, the combination of high anxiety, great expectations, and the up-and-down ride of cocaine was too much for his heart.

Dr. John Smialek, the Maryland Medical Examiner performed the autopsy on Bias.

It's not always possible when someone has a seizure and collapses to differentiate between a central nervous system stimulation for the seizure or an underlying cardiac event inducing the seizure. But in Bias's case it was pretty clear. His cardiac muscle showed a significant breakdown and inflammation. Now putting that evidence together with what we know about how cocaine affects the body, I concluded that the pathogenesis of this terminal event involved his heart directly and completely. Now the bigger question is, why did it happen to this man at this particular time, especially considering that we now know he used cocaine before? The only answer we can come up with at this time is that these things occur not randomly but when a person is especially susceptible. High susceptibility, though, depends on the nature of the person and his life at a given point of time.

To Smialek the Bias case is particularly disconcerting because it stirs up bad memories of an earlier investigation in which he participated. It shows, he says sadly, that regression — not progress — has occurred over the past ten years.

When Smialek was a medical investigator in the Pathology Department of the University of New Mexico at Albuquerque during the early 1980s, he and two colleagues encountered a troubling upswing in the number of youths suffering fatal cardiac arrest. They decided to examine these deaths more closely and discovered one crucial similarity linking them: in each case, the victim had inhaled typewriter correction fluid not long before his or her heart became arrhythmic. Though it may seem obvious today that drugs and arrhythmias are locked in a fatal bond, in 1980 they were considered entirely unconnected. At that time, tying drugs directly to heart arrhythmias seemed ridiculous to the medical community at large. But Smialek and his colleagues persisted with their research and, in effect, made the first cogent, evidentiary arguments that, without warning, drugs can cause immediate, irreversible cardiac arrest.

A typical case history from Smialek's New Mexico files is this gruesome story of a young girl.

A fourteen-year-old girl and her brother were sniffing white typewriter correction fluid (TCF) in their front yard with friends after being previously disciplined by their parents for engaging in such activity. The TCF was put into plastic bags and inhaled over a several-hour period. The deceased reportedly slumped over and was thought to have fallen asleep, and approximately thirty minutes passed before her brother realized she had stopped breathing. He summoned their parents, who initiated cardiopulmonary resuscitation. An ambulance was called but no heartbeat was found.

At the time of the autopsy, there was no external evidence of injury. Small flecks of white-colored adherent material was present on the back of the right thumb and the side and back of the right and left calves. (The deceased had been wearing shorts.)

Smialek says that the substance trichloroethylene is probably the cardiac killer in typewriter correction fluid, because it seems to exacerbate the natural arrhythmias caused by the body's production of adrenaline, which occurs in response to sniffing the drug.

And while, at that time, medical authorities agreed that the inhaling of trichloroethylene, as well as other aerosol products, often resulted in liver and kidney damage, what was most unusual about the cases we looked at was that no evidence of acute kidney and liver damage was exhibited. Instead, the circumstances suggested a sudden fatal cardiac arrhythmia as the mechanism of death.

Pressured by Smialek's study, public and private outcries, and the threat of suits, the manufacturers of typewriter correction fluid added warning labels to their products and even reformulated their recipes to include odorous, nontoxic agents — like mustard oil — to discourage intentional inhalation.

Unfortunately, Smialek's initial success in linking the social problem of drug abuse with the public health problem of arrhythmias has done little to curtail the number of deaths arising from drug-induced tachycardia and fibrillation. Indeed, the death of Len Bias made it painfully clear to him that not only has the problem not been eradicated, it has worsened. The stakes have risen as the drugs being consumed have become increasingly dangerous. Regretfully, Smialek says, what were once isolated incidents are now all too common and potentially lethal drugs like cocaine, heroin, and crack are widely disseminated among teenagers and even children.

I keep reliving the nightmare that the problem is probably more widespread than we recognize.

Steven Geevas, who treated Len Bias at Leland Memorial Hospital, concurs.

I've only been in the Emergency Room at this hospital for two years, but it seems monthly that I'm seeing younger and younger people come in here with cardiac arrest due to drugs.

Geevas feels that public education about the link between drugs and arrhythmias is the only solution, though virtually none is occurring despite the publicity surrounding Len Bias's death.

It's always a part of my treatment to educate my patients who suffer drug-related illnesses about what they're doing to themselves. Kids doing drugs have to realize that they're literally playing Russian roulette. There's a small margin that exists between euphoria and ventricular arrhythmia. And anyone can cross that threshold at any moment.

Geevas, though, is a realist — it's difficult to be anything else when you spend fifty to sixty hours a week treating people in an inner-city emergency room. He quickly concedes that patients who are panicking — still in the throes of a potentially devastating illness, vulnerable, and totally in the hands of physicians — promise the world to doctors. With religion in their eyes, they claim to have seen the light. Time, however, wears down their resolve. And long-term results, too often, are far less miraculous than their momentary "conversions."

Nine out of ten patients who come in after doing cocaine — who are on a bad trip and nearly didn't make it — tell you that they're quitting drugs for good. But who knows what they do next week when they're feeling immortal again. I have a feeling we lose a lot of them before long.

·10·

The First Line of Defense Against Arrhythmias: The Seattle Story

WHEN Jack W. walked briskly into the American Legion post in Ferndale, Washington, most of his colleagues were shocked to see him — and especially to see him looking so chipper. Just two weeks earlier, during a parade, he had lain prone, unconscious and apparently dying, on a rain-soaked street in nearby Seattle, a victim of sudden cardiac arrest. But a lightning response by the city's crack emergency medical system (EMS) team, the Medic 1 crew, and some of its residents turned a gruesome moment into a cause for celebration.

Put simply, Jack W. was lucky to collapse in Seattle, where saving patients dying from deadly arrhythmias is something of an art form. Indeed, nearly 400,000 residents of the city, 40 percent of the population, have been trained in cardiopulmonary resuscitation (CPR).

Seconds after a dizzy, nauseated, and dazed Jack W. passed out, several parade watchers administered CPR and others dialed the 911 emergency number. Three minutes later, firemen, trained as emergency medical technicians, were on the scene and took over the CPR effort, ensuring that at least a minimal amount of oxygen continued to course through Jack W.'s body, though his pulse had ceased because of ventricular fibrillation. In two more minutes, the Medic 1 group arrived. These cardiac technicians, with more than 1000 hours of advanced life-support studies under their belts, attached a portable defibrillator to Jack W.'s chest. Within seconds, his heart beat was returned to normal and he began to breathe on his own. In the ambulance, before he arrived at the Harborview Medical Center, the patient was conscious and alert. A week later, Jack W. was out of the hospital, back home in Ferndale and resuming the normal activities of his life.

This success story was possible because Jack W. was treated by an emergency medical team that is a true first line of defense against sudden cardiac death. Unfortunately, few other EMSs around the country are as enlightened as Seattle's in terms of understanding and treating arrhythmias. Though the obvious key to long-term treatment of a sudden cardiac arrest is ensuring that the patient arrives at the hospital alive, it is only very recently that an increasing number of EMSs in the United States have performed capably and consistently as the infantry in the battle against arrhythmias. In too many cases, the physicians in the electrophysiology labs are never given the opportunity to ply their clinical magic.

The soul of the Seattle emergency medical system attack against sudden cardiac arrest is Dr. Douglas Weaver, director of the Coronary Care Unit at Harborview Medical Center. Weaver, a quiet, confident physician, says that his interest in training EMS staff to understand and treat arrhythmias stems from one basic reality of modern cardiology: "You can't work in acute coronary care without realizing that the majority of the benefit which can be realized from a good emergency medical unit lies in its ability to thwart the syndrome of sudden cardiac death from serious ventricular arrhythmias."

Weaver adds that historically — and all too often today — emergency medical technicians and paramedics think of heart attack as a single illness, when, in reality, sudden cardiac arrest as a result of arrhythmias is frequently an entirely separate illness — and one especially worthy of focus by EMS squads.

In evaluations of patients who collapse suddenly with cardiac arrest outside the hospital, the proportion that are due to new heart attacks is relatively small, probably in the neighborhood of twenty-five percent. Instead, most patients who collapse unexpectedly have a sudden arrhythmia. They don't have a blockage of the coronary artery and a heart attack and then a subsequent arrhythmia. They simply have an unexplained arrhythmia that jolts them out of the blue.

In Weaver's view, assuming that a mobile coronary care unit or paramedic system is available, the chances of surviving a cardiac arrest when the EMS is aware of how to treat arrhythmias as opposed to when the emergency team is ignorant of the condition or ill-equipped to combat it, grow to about 30 percent from a woeful less than 5 percent.

Although more and more emergency medical teams are equipped with portable defibrillation devices and are becoming increasingly knowledgeable about the physiology of arrhythmias, the initial key to a patient's survival on the streets is the presence of a bystander able to initiate CPR. The EMS team is, at best, minutes away and each moment is critical. While waiting for the tools to be available to change the course of the arrhythmia, the patient whose pulse and breathing are seriously impaired must be supported by CPR.

"The paramedics can be carrying all the defibrillators in the world, but if CPR is delayed by more than a few minutes, the patient is unlikely to survive," says Weaver. "When a bystander initiates CPR at the scene prior to the arrival of the paramedic system, the plain fact is that the likelihood for that victim to live and to wake up with no functional impairment is substantially higher than if the first care received by that patient is initiated by an EMS team that has to travel to the emergency site."

However, Weaver adds, you usually can't do CPR for an extended period of time and expect a good outcome. A patient collapsed from an arrhythmia must be defibrillated within at least twelve minutes, usually closer to eight minutes, or his chances of regaining consciousness decline rapidly.

All of this was made clear during a study Weaver and his colleagues in Seattle conducted in 1986 of 251 patients who suffered sudden cardiac arrest due to arrhythmias. Forty-eight percent of the arrhythmia victims who received CPR in three minutes or less after collapsing survived, while only 36 percent lived after waiting more than three minutes before cardiopulmonary resuscitation was administered. Moreover, of those forty-four patients who lived after being given CPR during the first three minutes after arrest, 52 percent were defibrillated within six minutes, nearly 45 percent were defibrillated within seven to twelve minutes, and only 2 percent — one patient — survived when emergency cardiac care was more than twelve minutes away. Says Weaver:

> Analyzing this study as a whole and relating it to the times to beginning CPR and to initial defibrillation, mortality increased three percent each minute until CPR was begun and four percent a minute until the first shock was delivered.

Of course, necessity rules this scenario of CPR first and defibrillation second. Defibrillators are simply not available on every street corner and at every place people gather. But that's a tragically unfortunate reality, because while only 101, or 40 percent, of the 251 patients included in the Seattle study survived their attacks, it is estimated that as many as 188, or 75 percent, could have lived if defibrillators were immediately — that is, within seconds — on the scene.

"That's not just speculation," notes Dr. Leonard Cobb, professor of medicine at Seattle's University of Washington School of Medicine and a coauthor of the investigation. "In a cardiac rehabilitation program in the Seattle area there have been twenty-five cardiac arrests in patients who were undergoing supervised physical conditioning. Because defibrillators are immediately available in the rehab centers, each of these patients was successfully defibrillated, usually with only one shock."

The bottom line, then, is that by itself CPR rarely saves anybody's life. It's at best a holding measure. Unfortunately, there are still a lot of communities around the country that have only fire department or ambulance personnel — that is, basic emergency medical technicians, not cardiac crisis specialists — to administer CPR within the crucial first five minutes after collapse. The patient, then, has to be transported to a hospital fifteen minutes away or more for advanced care, such as defibrillation.

"That's not to say that under these systems someone isn't going to survive once in a while," says Cobb. "But I fear they survive despite the system rather than because of it."

It should be noted that while there has been a great deal of improvement in the availability of high-end emergency medical teams nationwide over the past few years, there has not been enough. In 1966, the National Highway Safety Act contained provisos that states upgrade their emergency medical services or lose 10 percent of their highway construction funds. Says Seattle cardiologist and arrhythmia specialist Dr. Mickey Eisenberg:

It's amazing to think of it this way, but twenty years ago prehospital emergency care was mainly given by poorly equipped private ambulances and mortuary companies, whose vehicles often doubled as hearses and whose personnel were only haphazardly trained in first aid.

Unfortunately, even faced with monetary penalties and a loss of road-construction grants, few states heeded the mandate of the 1966 Highway Act; this law had little effect on the dismal EMS capabilities of the United States. Then, in 1973, an Emergency Medical Systems Services law was passed. In this bill, the Department of Health, Education, and Welfare was given

$185 million to divide the nation into 300 emergency medical services regions that were to provide an integrated approach to EMS care. Today, fifteen years later, only one hundred of these regions are capable of on-site advanced life support with cardiac, trauma, neonatal, pediatric, and burn treatment facilities. The picture may be brighter, but clearly it is far from rosy.

The prototypical organizational structure for an EMS that specializes in thwarting sudden death from arrhythmias, as conceived by Douglas Weaver and his colleagues in Seattle over the past decade, is a multitiered operation.

It begins with having enough bystanders available who know how to perform CPR. In Seattle, the Medic II "civilian" CPR program is funded by the United Way, coordinated by the fire department, and is a well-publicized three-hour class. The fact that four out of ten residents of the metropolitan area have taken Medic II attests to the persistence and seriousness of the planners and students involved in this program.

The next tier are the first EMS responders — not the paramedics at the hospital. These EMS technicians must be local, within minutes of any critical medical situation. Call 911 in Seattle to report a cardiac arrest and dispatched to the scene are, simultaneously, emergency room paramedics and emergency medical staff from the nearest fire department trained in acute on-site coronary care, who can defibrillate and stabilize a patient before the hospital ambulance team arrives.

It wasn't always that way.

"In situations of cardiac arrest in the past, the firemen would only do CPR until the paramedics got there," says Weaver.

But realizing the great importance of this second, preparamedic, tier of emergency medical support, in the early 1980s Weaver worked with a local clinical equipment manufacturer, Physio-Control Corporation, to design an automatic, fifteen-pound, portable defibrillator — known as the Lifepak. The machine is akin to the large devices that shock hearts into normal rhythms in hospitals all over the world. The main difference is that the portable unit analyzes for the emergency medical technician whether an arrhythmia is present and then advises whether defibrillation should be performed or not. Instead of the relatively complicated devices used in hospital labs, which require a fair amount of training in reading the heart's condition from the electrocardiograph and oscilloscopes, the Lifepak can be used by any minimally trained lay person.

Soon after its completion, Weaver tested the device in life and death situations.

We gave the Lifepak to the first responding firefighters in our tiered emergency medical system and authorized them to use the device until the paramedics arrived on the scene. They could deliver shocks as well as CPR. A quarter of the people that were treated with the Lifepak had regained pulse and circulation and some were even awake by the time the paramedics arrived. This was an unusual, unprecedented statistic. By chopping off a few minutes for defibrillation, it appeared we had a device that potentially could have an extremely significant impact on emergency cardiac care.

To use the Lifepak, the firefighter rapidly examines the victim to determine that a cardiac arrest is present and then applies self-adhesive paddles containing monitoring and defibrillation electrodes to the chest. He then presses the "Analyze" button on the Lifepak. Second laters, after the device examines the EKG for an arrhythmia, a message is displayed on the unit's screen, either "Shock Advised" or "No Shock Advised." If the former appears, the firefighter pushes the Lifepak's "Shock" button and the patient is defibrillated with a 200-joule dose of electricity.

Steven S. owes his life to the Lifepak. He experienced five separate cardiac arrests in his home and survived each of them for one reason: he lives next-door to the fire station and the portable defibrillator.

Forty-seven-year-old Simon A.'s bout with sudden death from arrhythmia was more touch and go than any of Steven S.'s.

One rainy morning, he was shopping in an outdoor farm market when he collapsed suddenly. His friend immediately began administering CPR, while a bystander reported the medical emergency to the EMS by dialing 911. The nearest firefighters were there in less then three minutes, attached the Lifepak to his chest, and defibrillated his out-of-synch heart. By the time the paramedics arrived, three minutes later, Simon A. was fully awake and alert.

The paramedics inserted an IV cannula into Simon A.'s arm in order to have an emergency line to administer drugs on the way to the hospital should it be necessary. No breathing tube was put into his trachea.

But nothing untoward happened during the ambulance ride, and later that day Simon A. left the hospital feeling fit. (Follow-up sessions were scheduled for the next couple of weeks to determine how to treat the arrhythmia.) One of the paramedics, describing this case, adds:

> Having the fireman use the portable defibrillator changes the whole ballgame. Previously, I would be responsible for taking care of the heart rhythms while my partner had to work on putting a tube down the patient's trachea for oxygen and an IV in his body for drugs. Meanwhile, during all of this the patient is still on the ground, precious time is being wasted before we can begin to carry him to the hospital. Usually, you have to be prepared for the worst. Now, with more and more situations like this occurring, where the patient is already stable when we arrive and we only have to get the patient into the ambulance, we can be prepared for the best. And this really changes the outcome for people.

Simon A.'s case is somewhat uncommon. More frequently, even after the arrhythmia is reversed by the firefighters, the patient does not immediately regain consciousness. So during the trip to the hospital the paramedics must administer drugs and oxygen through tubes. Meanwhile, an electrocardiograph continues to monitor the patient's heart and transmit the results to the emergency room, while a two-way radio enables the physicians at the hospital to hear and respond to the survival efforts in progress. Thus, nearly all in-ambulance therapy is carried out in consultation with the emergency room staff.

"On the average," notes Weaver, "with this system the paramedics are successful sixty percent of the time in restoring pulse and blood pressure and bringing the patient into the hospital in a conscious state."

If there is one disconcerting failing of the Seattle EMS program it is that a very important part of the population has not taken the Medic II CPR classes. By and large, the cardiopulmonary resuscitation training has been attended by younger men. But significantly, elderly women have generally stayed away from the classes. Says Weaver:

> This is of particular concern, because arrhythmias — and heart disease, in general — occur in elderly men. Moreover, frequently the attack occurs at home. So you'd want the older women to be trained in CPR. Perhaps we as physicians should become more involved and stress to those people who have family members that are at greatest risk for sudden cardiac arrest that they must be trained in CPR to save the lives of their loved ones.

·11·

On Walton's Mountain

I N the mid-1970s, Dr. Richard Crampton was a young Southern physician with a dream, though many in those days refused to dignify his notion with such an epithet. Instead, it was
called an utterly wasteful medical experiment by one former
colleague. Another put it more bluntly: "You can't teach un-
schooled rednecks to do the work of doctors."

Yet, that was exactly what Crampton had in mind. As director of the Coronary Care Unit at the University of Virginia
Medical Center in Charlottesville — the "big" city where the
buses, courthouses, and specialist physicians could be found in
the television show "The Waltons" — the now forty-five-year-
old doctor knew he had to do something to upgrade the ability
of the hospital's EMS to deal with arrhythmia attacks. Either
that or cave in to the thought that saving the lives of cardiac
arrest victims in wide-open rural spaces is an impossible task.

The University of Virginia hospital is one of the few teaching
medical centers in the United States located out in the country — Dartmouth, in rural New Hampshire, is another prominent example. The University of Virginia hospital has a

surrounding community of 80,000 people spread out over 745 mountainous square miles. The acres and acres of hardwoods and pine bluffs covering thousands of tons of coal and granite make the terrain particularly difficult to negotiate quickly for ambulances and physicians racing to patients. Indeed, many of the patients served by the hospital are as distant as fifty miles — or over an hour — away.

What is more, in 1970, when Crampton decided to look at the situation closely, responding to this far-flung rural region was an EMS woefully ill-equipped to deal with cardiac emergencies. Hardly anybody manning the ambulances was trained in CPR, few could read an EKG, and none could operate a defibrillator. In short, a collapsed patient stricken by an arrhythmia in the Charlottesville hills would not only have to wait a long time before the EMS arrived, but could expect only a ride to the hospital with no medical care after the ambulance drove up.

"It may have been a good taxi service, but it didn't offer what anybody in his right mind could call anything near an acceptable clinical response," says Crampton.

Perhaps the most telling statistic for the inability of the University of Virginia EMS to treat coronary patients is the one that describes the number of patients saved who suffered cardiac emergencies en route to the hospital. Put simply, in this regard the performance of the University of Virginia EMS could not have been worse.

"No number has yet been discovered lower than zero," Crampton explains, "and that's exactly how many people the ambulance corps saved from death by sudden cardiac arrest in their vehicles from 1966 through 1970."

In those five years, the University of Virginia EMS team put into their ambulances eighty-three ill people who were unexpectedly stricken by cardiac arrhythmias while riding to the hospital. Not once did it bring one of those patients in alive. Crampton found this figure to be the ultimate metaphor for how badly the University of Virginia emergency coronary medical care system operated.

Crampton decided to eradicate this woeful inadequacy with one swift move. In early 1971, he equipped his EMS team with its initial array of prehospital emergency cardiac equipment, including a portable suction apparatus — a device that keeps the airway open after a patient vomits during cardiac arrest or a seizure — an electrocardiograph, and a defibrillator. At the same time he hired additional emergency room staff and trained them in out-of-hospital life-support techniques. For the first time, the University of Virginia had a mobile coronary care unit.

And the turnaround was stunning. In 1971, twenty patients suffered cardiac arrests in the ambulance; four survived. In 1972, fifteen were stricken en route; nine survived. And in 1973, eleven patients went into arrest while being rushed to the hospital; the EMS recorded seven saves.

In Crampton's mind he had performed a minor medical miracle — but it was not enough. Despite the vast improvement in the EMS team's performance when victims were stricken in their ambulances, those victims who were stricken before the ambulance arrived and survived the trip to the hospital were still few and far between. Accurate statistics were not kept, but it is estimated that, at most, 1 percent of all those who collapsed from arrhythmias in their home or in the streets of the Charlottesville area during the early 1970s were revived for the trip to the University of Virginia hospital.

The endemic problem was clear to Crampton. Though well-equipped for cardiac care now, the University of Virginia EMS simply could not get to most areas of the hospital's communities in time to resuscitate arrhythmia victims. Short of flattening the mountains and building a network of modern roads, nothing could be done to diminish the cardiac death rate in the hills and hollows. And it was in this context that by the late 1970s Crampton came up with the idea that was initially so maligned: if the existing emergency medicine system could not reach the rural communities in time, he reasoned, why not turn each of the rural communities into an EMS.

"It was an outlandish notion," says Diana Rockwell, the

critical care nurse chosen by Crampton for the "impossible" task of training the small-town, country rescue squads in the techniques of the most sophisticated, prehospital cardiac care.

And she told Crampton this during their first meeting, when he proposed that she take on the job of heading this new EMS program.

"There's no way I can teach these poorly educated, back-woods people how to resuscitate the cardiac dead," Rockwell said, questioning in her mind Crampton's sanity in even con-juring up such a scheme. "They don't even know what an EKG is. How can they possibly learn to analyze one?"

Crampton looked at her with a frozen, steadfast stare, un-moved by her pessimism. He said quietly: "I don't care how long it takes you, if they want to be taught, you teach them. The only requirement that I've put on the trainees is they have a high school diploma."

Beyond training, there was another obstacle to be overcome in order to put Crampton's plan into operation. The rural res-cue squads had to be convinced that they needed to be outfitted for prehospital cardiac care. Actually that wasn't very difficult. Considering their failure in treating arrhythmia victims, little pressure had to be put on the rescue teams before they realized the necessity to upgrade their response to cardiac patients.

But these groups were financially strapped, relying on cake sales, fireworks displays, and donations solicited door-to-door to keep their small-scale, simple operations alive. None could afford the $60,000 it would cost to "go cardiac." Eyeing the list of equipment that they had to purchase — an electrocar-diograph and monitor; a defibrillator; a telemetry unit to send heart rhythms information to the University of Virginia emer-gency room so that a physician could monitor the in-the-field cardiac crisis and offer assistance; a base station at the hospital to receive this data; and an ambulance large enough for tech-nicians to stand up in — the rescue squads begged off the proj-ect, pleading poverty.

Crampton was undaunted. A directed effort enabled him to

wrest over a quarter of a million dollars from the federal Emergency Medical Systems Services legislation to upgrade the rural emergency teams. Crampton then set up a grant arrangement in which he paid 100 percent the first year and 25 percent less each succeeding year to aid the squads. The rural groups pitched in with a high-gear campaign to get increased donations from their communities. The entire effort payed off handsomely. By 1983, all seven regional rescue groups in the Charlottesville area were equipped for prehospital cardiac care.

In the meantime, Diana Rockwell began to train the would-be cardiac technicians in emergency coronary medical care. It was an ambitious program by any standards. First, trainees had to take a quarter-year Shock Trauma course that consisted of three-hour classes twice a week and then twenty-four more hours working in the emergency room with an instructor. During these sessions, they learned to recognize and evaluate the critically ill and injured and how to initiate treatments.

After they passed this course, the trainees were given the Cardiac Technician classes. During another three months of sessions, they were taught the nature and makeup of the cardiac patient; how to read and interpret EKGs; analysis of arrhythmias, including which are life threatening and which are benign; and the techniques for treating dysrhythmias. Rockwell explains:

> Our goal is to teach the trainees how to put what they are observing about the patient and the patient's EKG together. That is crucial to developing competent cardiac technicians. One thing you have to break people of is the habit of relying too strongly on the EKG and interpreting it without also assessing the patient. Some people can have dreadful EKGs but be healthy and happy. This is because electrocardiograph leads can come off or the machine may be malfunctioning. If EKGs are the sole criteria for emergency cardiac care there can be an awful lot of unnecessary defibrillation.

In all, since the training program started, Rockwell has graduated nearly two hundred cardiac technicians. This is remarkable in light of the fact that many of the students work a hard forty hours each week and often commute an hour to get to the classes. What's more, a significant amount of homework and studying are required between training sessions.

One of my favorite students was a woodcutter who put his EKG analyses on little cards in his pocket. When his son was driving the timber to market, he sat on a stump and studied EKGs. He doesn't know how to say lidocaine or epinephrine — he pronounces it epiephrine — but he can revive a person who has collapsed from sudden cardiac arrest.

Saving lives is a bug that these volunteers catch and once they're into the EMT system they want to get all that they can out of it. In fact, what happens often is that they burn themselves out. They end up having to run over to neighbors' houses to sort through real or imagined illnesses even if they're not on duty.

Though Rockwell's training has earned high marks, a large number of medical professionals in the Charlottesville area continue to naysay and mock the rural rescue squad cardiac treatment plan.

Explains Rockwell: "This is a conservative community and they have a hard time with nonprofessionals or people outside of their immediate system performing things like defibrillating a dying patient. They've even told me, 'My God, shocking a patient! My nurses aren't even allowed to do that.' This is very, very terrifying and frightening for them."

Crampton's response: "Shoot, what do you have to lose?"

Actually, it's what they have to save that is so precious. And no one knows this better than Jim S., the seventeen-year-old black track star who was jogging at his high school track in the distant hills twenty miles from Charlottesville. Suddenly, the teenager dropped, unconscious. A physical education teacher ran toward the stricken youth from a nearby dugout where he was going over student test scores.

He shook Jim S. a few times, saw he was unconscious, and initiated cardiopulmonary resuscitation. Meanwhile, he yelled to a student on the far turn of the track: "Call 911, quick! Tell them we've got a heart attack!"

The teacher kept pouring air into Jim S.'s lungs and compressing his heart, but the youngster was barely alive. He was not breathing and had no pulse.

The local rescue squad, one of Crampton's cardiac units, arrived within five minutes. The emergency technician immediately put the electrocardiograph paddles on Jim S. and with the first line of read-out on the monitor saw the unmistakable wavering, patternless spikes of ventricular fibrillation. The tech then attached defibrillator electrodes to Jim S.'s chest and shocked the track star with 200 joules of electricty.

Jim S.'s body arched in the shape of an inverted U, the small of his back shooting skyward. Then he relaxed again. The cardiac technician looked quickly at the electrocardiograph monitor. In that one jolt, Jim S.'s heart rhythms had returned to normal. His breathing was still labored, so the rescue squad chief put an oxygen tube down his airway. Further, to thwart any new arrhythmias he injected the drug lidocaine through an intravenous line.

Still unconscious, but stable, Jim S. was put into the ambulance and the vehicle began speeding toward the hospital, nearly twenty minutes away. During the drive to the hospital, emergency room physicians at the University of Virginia monitored the patient's EKG and vital signs through the ambulance's telemetry unit. As far as the physicians were concerned, the EMS unit could not have performed any better. Indeed, just a few moments before the ambulance arrived at the hospital, Jim S. regained consciousness. He was lethargic but was now out of immediate danger.

Relieved by Jim S.'s sudden turn for the better, the physicians at the University of Virginia, sounding like ground control after just talking astronauts through a tough landing, congratulated the rescue squad on a job well done. The EMTs were told to bypass the emergency room and bring Jim S. directly to the coronary care unit.

Jim S., it turns out, was suffering from a disease known as IHSS, in which the ventricles enlarge and obstruct the flow of blood into the aorta. In turn, cardiac rhythms are undermined. About one third of all patients with IHSS have had the condition since birth, while many of the other victims develop the disease over many years for reasons that are at present unknown.

In Jim S.'s case he crossed over both categories. He had a congenitally thickened left ventricle, which hypertrophied even more with his constant athletic training. Placed on a regimen of drugs to reduce the cardiac hypertrophy, Jim S. was almost immediately able to return to his previous life-style.

It is case histories like this one, says Diana Rockwell, that constantly reaffirm her belief that Richard Crampton's rural emergency medicine concept is tinged with brilliance.

I mean Jim S. should have been dead, plain and simple. We had the exact same situation at another county high school before the rescue squads were equipped with electrocardiographs and defibrillators — then they could only do CPR — and the patient died. I have never seen any arrhythmia victim from a rural area or an urban area that has lived after only receiving CPR before reaching the hospital.

Perhaps the hardest part of the volunteer cardiac technician's job is that under pressure — with a stricken person lying there who will be unrevivable in a matter of minutes — he has to recall, without slipping, the meaning of different EKGs, the correct treatments and drug dosages for vastly dissimilar cardiac treatments, and how to use equipment that is too frequently uncooperative. With life and death hanging in a scale that is growing more and more unbalanced by the second, the cardiac technician has one choice and it must be the right one. His decisions, made without consulting a physician, have no built-in fail-safe valves.

Still the best cardiac technicians are confident, even cocky, about how they handled the last emergency and are poised for the next one.

In most instances, when we go over their work, the techs are steadfast in the conviction that they wouldn't do anything differently. Look, if you want to compare a physician to a volunteer cardiac tech, I'll take the cardiac tech any day in a life-threatening situation. They've been drilled and drilled and drilled as to how to act in any given emergency situation. The physician may have forgotten all he's learned about emergency medicine by now. Physicians feel the same way. It's not unusual for a physician to be at the scene of a cardiac arrest and say to the techs, "You guys supervise here. Tell me what to do and I'll do it." You can imagine that when a rural tech hears this — when a woodcutter or a mechanic or a mason or even a nurse hears a physician talking to him like this — it's pretty exciting. It's also incredibly scary.

Diana Rockwell knows first-hand how it feels to lead an emergency cardiac resuscitation effort when a physician pleads ignorance and takes the back seat. It was a complicated case with failure written all over it — and it's one that she will never forget. In her career, it's the patient who got away — and shouldn't have.

The story is of twenty-one-year-old Emily K., a young woman from the hollows of Virginia who lived in nearly abject poverty and had little medical care throughout her life. On a windy, stormy night, when the thunder cracked like butting moose-heads and lightning lit up the soft green hills with jagged flashes, Emily K. and her mother walked to the local lodge for weekly bingo.

The game was only about ten minutes old when Emily K. felt a sharp twinge pierce her chest. A mere five minutes later, she collapsed. Chaos ensued. Some people screamed; others ran over to Emily K.'s stricken body and started loosening her clothing, while the bingo caller dialed the 911 emergency line and reported a cardiac emergency. The hall was filled with women, and this emergency served as an unfortunate reminder that few women take CPR lessons. Nobody in the room was capable of performing cardiopulmonary resuscitation on Emily K. So it seemed, at least.

Unbeknownst to anybody else at the lodge that night, in the middle of the panic and the tumult, the fifteen-year-old retarded son of Mrs. J., seated at the back of the room, was about to come forward and give CPR to the arrhythmia victim. The youth had learned CPR with his father, who was a local rescue squad worker. But his mother restrained him. She stared straight into her boy's eyes and shook her head firmly.

Mrs. J. recalls that moment ruefully. It still gives her chills to think about what she did as her son was about to get up. But she says that she wouldn't do anything differently today.

> I know it sounds cruel, but I had no choice. If my son failed to save her life, he would have been blamed unmercifully. He's suffering enough, being retarded and all, that I couldn't risk him suffering any more emotional pain. I'm not saying he would've failed, but I simply couldn't risk it. It may sound crazy to outsiders, but I know my neighbors and I know what people would have said about my son.

With nobody available to perform CPR, Emily K. was clearly dying. The EMTs arrived about eight minutes after she collapsed. When the call came in of the cardiac emergency, the closest rescue group was a cardiac technician class being taught by Diana Rockwell. So the entire group went to the lodge to treat the stricken woman.

"For my students it was baptism under fire, for me it was

not much better," recalls Rockwell. "Especially when the lights went out."

Just as Rockwell and her group arrived, the battering storm shorted out all of the electricity in the area. They were forced to treat Emily K. in the dark, under the illumination of small flashlights.

> We did what we could under the circumstances. One of my team began immediate CPR and another defibrillated without delay, primarily because it was clear from her dangerously low pulse rate that she had been arrhythmic for some time. I didn't want to take the time to try to read the EKGs in the dim light.

In the meantime, Rockwell called a nearby doctor who she knew had a generator in her office. Rockwell asked the physician to get her electricity operating because they were bringing a patient in. Defibrillation and CPR had stabilized Emily K. somewhat — her pulse was steadier and she was beginning to breathe on her own. But she was clearly in need of an immediate drug regimen, and Rockwell feared that her heart might fibrillate again before long. They put Emily K. into the ambulance and had her on the doctor's table, under full overhead lights, in less than a minute.

Rockwell was relieved when Emily K. was in the physician's office. All of the tension dissipated. The patient, she thought, was now the physician's concern — and that is as it should be. The emergency squad was only a Band-Aid, not a cure. At least, that's what her schooling and experience had taught her. But that night she learned differently.

Rockwell turned to the doctor and pointed to the patient. "Thank the Lord that you're here. We've already performed CPR and defibrillated her. But she's still in very dangerous territory."

The physician looked at Rockwell quizzically. "Don't let me get in your way. You seem to have it under control. Go ahead and tell me what to do."

Recalls Rockwell:

I didn't say anything to the doctor, but inside I was screaming, "Oh, no, don't put that responsibility on me." In the next thought, though, I realized something else. That physician's reaction told me how important the cardiac teams had become for this region and how ignorant so many doctors are about emergency prehospital cardiac care.

Rockwell pulled out all the stops and stabilized Emily K. — although it was an uneasy equilibrium that she settled into — for the long, fifty-mile trip to the University of Virginia hospital. But that was to be Emily K.'s last trip through the narrow, unforgiving roads of the back hills of Virginia. Two days later she died. Rockwell rues Emily K.'s story even in the telling.

She was so long without oxygen that she was irrevocably damaged. You can't wait eight minutes before initiating CPR and expect a patient to survive. Unfortunately, though, Emily K.'s story is all too typical for our area. The truth of our cardiac emergency medical system is that we can save, at most, 10 percent of the patients that collapse from arrhythmias out of the hospital. If you provide CPR within four to six minutes and get the EMS there within eight minutes, you'll save 50 percent of the victims. Sadly, most of the time we are unable to meet that timetable.

But there is something even more important to say about Emily K. She wouldn't have died if she had proper medical care during her life. She was suffering from a congenital condition of the heart. The doctors should have been aware of it, because her brother had died a few years earlier of the very same birth defect. But nobody ever examined her after her brother's death for this problem. She was poor, and the extent of her medical care was backwood clinics. I guess she fell through the cracks of the county's medical system.

Because time is so utterly crucial in an arrhythmia crisis, emergency medical specialists are pressing rural, suburban, and urban communities to implement more and more sophisticated communications networks for reporting a cardiac collapse and ensuring that the rescue team quickly knows the location of the victim. Though some areas are still without a "911" system — a short, easy-to-remember telephone number to dial when notifying the police, ambulance, and fire departments of an emergency — EMS squads already consider 911 obsolete and are recommending something known as "enhanced 911." With enhanced 911, a computer automatically logs in the exact site of the emergency the moment the phone call reporting it is received. Rescue squads can be dispatched immediately to the victim's side without waiting for the caller to spell out the address; addresses, it has been shown time and time again, are difficult to remember when a loved one is in serious danger of dying.

And enhanced 911 has an additional benefit as a crime stopper. In urban areas like New York City where, authorities claim, up to 50 percent of all emergency calls to the 911 line are false alarms, no longer are the locations of the criminals taking up the EMS's time shielded in anonymity.

But 911 or enhanced 911 is useless unless houses are posted with large, easy-to-find street-number signs — either on the mailbox, porch columns, or the front door — that stand out at all hours of the day and night and that are not hidden by dense foliage during the spring and summer. This is particularly a problem in less-populated rural areas where, sadly, it is not uncommon for ambulance drivers to ride through complicatedly interwoven back roads for several damaging minutes — the absolute difference between life and death — because the house they're looking for and those around it are unmarked.

The overt fear and disrespect that initially greeted Richard Crampton's extremely successful country cardiac rescue squads is not unusual for rural areas; its goes to the heart of what the citizens of the nation's small towns see the role of an EMS to be — and it's in sharp contrast to the emergency medicine expectations of city dwellers. Urban areas view emergency medicine as a birthright. EMTs are expected to save lives — anyone's — at all costs. One EMT at San Francisco General Hospital recalls that in the predefibrillator days of the early 1970s, when heart thumping, cardiac massage, and CPR was all a coronary victim could expect, derelicts from the Mission District who went into cardiac arrest would be revived and then die repeatedly — sometimes twenty to thirty times — until the rescue workers' arms and lungs ached from the back-breaking and muscle-taxing effort. The clear mandate that EMSs hew to in the cities is that death is only given into after a long, numbing struggle. But in rural areas, the attitude towards death is vastly different — there death is accepted far more stoically and is often seen as God's messenger calling the victim home — and the EMTs are forced to perform with this attitude in mind.

This divergence of EMS philosophies, urban versus rural, was hammered home not long ago when Crampton raised the difficult question at an emergency medicine seminar, "Is pre-hospital cardiac life support ever a violation of a person's right to die with dignity?"

Leonard Cobb, of the University of Washington School of Medicine at Seattle and one of the architects of that city's excellent emergency medical system, thought Crampton's query did not apply to the actions of a cardiac EMT.

> Whether or not to initiate basic cardiac life support may be a difficult decision outside the hospital, because you usually don't know the patient's medical history. But if we're called to a cardiac arrest, we'll always attempt to resuscitate the patient. We can't make "no code" judgments on the basis of a ten-second examination. We assume when someone calls it's for good reason. What do you do?

Crampton said that the way the University of Virginia's EMS regards the situation could not be more different because it confronts a sharply contrasting social environment.

With only 40,000 folks in the city of Charlottesville and 80,000 in all of the communities in our region, we're vastly smaller than Seattle, and maybe everybody knows each other a little better than Seattle. It's not uncommon for the squad to call in and say, "Look, we're at the home of Mrs. Brown. She's apparently suffered cardiac arrest. A family friend called us in but now her son is here, and he says his mother's got terminal cancer." In a situation like that it would be a charade to continue CPR and bring the patient into the emergency room.

I've also been in situations in particularly touch-and-go cases where I've had to tell the unit personnel to terminate the cardiac arrest procedure because the mobile unit was forty-five minutes away from the nearest hospital. We'd be asking the emergency personnel to continue basic cardiac life support in an ambulance on a winding country road for about an hour's time on a patient who probably won't survive anyway. That's not pleasant but it does happen.

In his environment, Crampton adds, medical miracles are fleeting, God's aren't. Though he has spent his recent professional years turning uncomplicated people, who live simply and unostentatiously, into skilled cardiac technicians, he knows that in the end his success depends entirely on how well he supports the often religious notions that guide the day-to-day existence of his constituency, not on attempting to change these ideas.

·12·

The Electronic Security Blanket

THERE'S an old wives' tale, ironically probably promulgated by men, that as soon as you retire you begin to die. The body, which seemed so invincible and unbreakable during the virile working years, just can't seem to take the strain of enforced relaxation. Some dismiss this notion as pure superstition, but don't try to convince Robert H. of that. He believes that he's living proof of it.

For nearly fifty years, Robert H. owned an auto parts outlet in the center of Washington's Skagit River Valley, a rich, bucolic farm region, where, as he describes it, "vehicles are pushed to the limit and break down about as often as weeds need picking." The parts store prospered, though it demanded long hours of back-breaking attention. Finally, at age seventy, coaxed by his wife, Denise, Robert H. sold the shop and retired.

Six months later, while sitting on his back porch staring at the tulips and raspberries that covered the hills towering over the valley, Robert H. suddenly suffered a warningless, symptomless cardiac arrest. Slowly and silently — almost in slow motion — he fell to the floor.

Denise heard him tumble out of his chair. She ran out of the house to find him unconscious and gasping. Screaming for help, she rushed across the street to a neighbor who was a former nurse. Cardiopulmonary resuscitation was performed and Robert H. was revived. A half-an-hour later, Robert H. was lying in a bed at the local hospital with tubes, catheters, and a respirator crisscrossing his body.

Mt. Vernon is a rural medical center without the medical equipment or staff to treat a complicated case of cardiac arrest. Still, Robert H. was put through a battery of tests over the next week-and-a-half that seemed to point to nothing conclusive as the cause of his collapse. Unsure how to proceed, Robert H.'s physicians suggested that he go to Harborview Hospital in nearby Seattle for further analysis.

Fortunately, because Robert H.'s sudden cardiac arrest was brought on by a cardiac arrhythmia, Harborview is one of the premier electrophysiology centers in the country. In an effort to find the right anti-arrhythmia pharmacological strategy for Robert H. — if there was one — the physicians in Seattle administered various drugs, then tried to reinduce the arrhythmia in the electrophysiology lab. The first two drugs failed to stem the arrhythmia. But finally, the third, Amiodarone, did and two per day were prescribed.

Robert H. was also told to take home something else besides the pills: a portable defibrillator. As one of his cardiologists explains:

> We've learned by now that drugs are simply not a final solution for arrhythmias. But if no arrhythmia is inducible in the electrophysiology lab after a patient has been given a large dose of a particular drug, we're constrained to prescribe it. That doesn't allay our doubts and our concerns, but we're forced to prescribe it. We cannot ethically perform an invasive procedure when a noninvasive treatment like a pharmacological one has already passed the test. So it's comforting to send the patient home with a portable defibrillator — an if-I-fall-over-dead-please-put-

this-on-my-chest-and-go-zap sort of device. At least it gives the patient a security blanket that I believe the drugs don't provide.

The portable defibrillator that left the hospital with Robert H. was about the size of a shoe box and weighed a little over six pounds. It essentially performs the same functions as the large defibrillators in coronary care units and electrophysiology labs and the slightly smaller defibrillators carried by emergency medical teams — with a streak of electricity, a countershock, it normalizes the pulse of an arrhythmic heart — but the difference is, it, and not a doctor or a cardiac technician, makes the decision whether to defibrillate or not. When its paddles are placed on a collapsed patient's chest, the portable defibrillator analyzes the patient's condition and advises on the proper course of action. If defibrillation is called for, the patient's partner presses a SHOCK button and the machine administers the counterjolt.

Robert H. and Denise were skeptical about this new unit, which was supposed to become an inseparable companion.

"Old-timers like us are not comfortable with complicated-looking machines that you take home and administer to yourself," says Denise. "That's not what we're used to medicine being all about."

But a few months later, at Christmastime, Robert H. and his wife found out that their skepticism toward the portable defibrillator was unfounded. Luckily, they had not heeded their initial negative feelings toward the device.

They were traveling in their recreational vehicle to Anaheim in Southern California to visit their children for the holidays. It was dusk in the Central Valley when the fog poured in unexpectedly and relentlessly; suddenly, visibility was reduced to two feet at its best moments. Deciding not to risk an accident, the couple pulled into a truck-stop parking lot and stayed there through the night.

The next morning — early, not much past six — Robert H. and Denise ate breakfast and then got back into the RV to proceed south. But as Robert H. turned the key in the van, sparks flew from under the hood. A slight electrical short set off a small, contained fire in the engine. Robert H. and Dorothy ran out of the RV. He opened the hood quickly, while she rushed to the back of the van to grab the fire extinguisher. Staring down into the engine and realizing that his holiday vacation had effectively been short-circuited, Robert H. was angry and frustrated. As the tension rose sweat covered him, needling him like bursts of prickly heat.

> I guess I got overexcited. My heart began to pound and kick my chest from inside and out. I began to get dizzy and lose my balance. Just before I fell over I steadied myself on the grill of the mobile home for a second. I remember that and then I remember nothing. I passed out.

Fortunately for Robert H., while Denise was not completely convinced that the portable defibrillator would be of real value, she had followed the rules of thumb for it recommended by the trainers at Harborview.

> They told me to always put the defibrillator in the same easy-to-reach place and to always put it back there. This way, like second nature, I'd know where to grab for it when I needed it.

Panicking somewhat, but controlled enough to know that the only chance she had of saving her husband's life was to follow the step-by-step procedures for using the portable defibrillator, Denise reached into the van next to the luggage and pulled the device out. She opened the box that held the portable defibrillator and put the paddles on Robert H.'s chest. As she describes it:

> It took two breaths of CPR, then one shock from the portable defibrillator, then more CPR and I could see him starting to breathe on his own.

A minute later, Robert H. was completely recovered from his bout with cardiac arrest from arrhythmia. He looked up at Denise, his eyes wide open. A confused look spread across his face. "What happened?"

"Those were really good words for me to hear at that point," says Denise.

"I could've easily stood up and walked away," Robert H. adds. Instead, following the rules of the rescue team, which had been summoned by a bystander and arrived moments later, Robert H. was taken to the local hospital. He was released after a day of cardiac monitoring and no additional signs of heart problems. They continued their trip to Anaheim.

What is most dramatic about the case of Robert H. is the unforgettable fact that had he not been treated at Harborview Hospital, where arrhythmias are not a foreign concept, he would not be alive today. There are few cardiologists in the United States who have even heard of a portable defibrillator and fewer still with the imagination to prescribe one.

Although it is a new and virtually untried procedure, out-of-hospital defibrillation is saving lives. It may be the most crucial prescription for diminishing the unacceptable mortality rates from arrhythmias, both for those patients who have already suffered one sudden cardiac arrest and those who are stricken with it suddenly, with no symptomatic warnings. Notes Jeremy Ruskin:

> The key to releasing the lethal grip that arrhythmias have on the overall populace is putting inexpensive, portable, easily operated defibrillators in every dormitory, airplane, restaurant, hotel, school, stadium, etc. — in any location where large numbers of people live or congregate — and training people to use them.

Though it is occurring slowly, the call for portable defibrillators in public places is being heeded in at least a few quarters. British Caledonian, the international airline, for instance, is carrying a portable defibrillator on many of its international routes to evaluate their effectiveness. Manning the portable defibrillators is a new breed of flight attendant, an aviation medical technician (AMT). The AMTs are actually cardiac emergency medical staffers who are trained to analyze passenger emergencies, operate a portable defibrillator, and inject anti-arrhythmic medications for short-term survival — that is, until the plane is down and the patient can get to a hospital.

One important by-product of the portable defibrillators for the nation's health care system is that it allows patients to be sent home far sooner than before, providing a potential savings of millions of dollars each year on physicians' bills and hospitalization costs. Dr. Bruce Goldreyer, associate professor of medicine at the University of Southern California and director of Diagnostic Cardiology at San Pedro Peninsula Hospital, lays out the scenario:

> In terms of overall cardiac care you save substantial money by sending people home earlier with a portable defibrillator. After treatment for a myocardial infarct [a typical arrhythmia-causing cardiac condition in which sections of the heart muscle die and scar due to a lack of blood to the region], for example, instead of sending the patient home on the tenth or twelfth day, you could release him on the fifth day and feel pretty secure that, if an arrhythmia occurs, at least the patient can be defibrillated at home and live long enough to get back to the hospital. Look, the twelfth-day release notion is not a scientific concept anyway; I've had patients who go home after twelve days and die from a cardiac arrest on the thirteenth.
>
> What's more, some antiarrhythmic drugs take six weeks to "load" into the body, when you can really be sure that it is going to be effective, for a while at least. But it's unreasonable to keep them in the hospital for that long. So you have to send them out of here unprotected. You're caught between a rock and a hard place in your management of the patient. The portable defibrillator gives you

an alternative therapy for these patients. That is, you've got the comfort of them being at home, and yet you have the safety factor — the knowledge that you've given them the means to be defibrillated should something occur.

The two leading portable defibrillators are Lifepak 100, from Physio-Control Corporation (Redmond, Washington) and Heart*Aid, manufactured by Cardiac Resuscitator Corporation (Portland, Washington). These battery-powered units operate similarly, but differ in two distinct ways. At twenty pounds and the size of *two* shoe boxes, Heart*Aid is quite a bit larger than the diminutive, six-pound Lifepak 100, the device that defibrillated Robert H. during his trip to Southern California. But for the extra bulk of Heart*Aid, there is a premium: unlike Lifepak 100, it requires no assistance from bystanders or the patient's partner; instead, once it is activated, Heart*Aid automatically analyzes and then shocks the patient's heart, if necessary.

Reading a transcript of a session in which a portable defibrillator is used to resuscitate a collapsed patient is like being immersed in the climax of a fiction thriller. You can almost hear the clock ticking mercilessly as the portable defibrillator races against time to sort out the subtle and outwardly inscrutable dimensions of the cardiac crisis and revive a near-dead person.

ELAPSED TIME

00:00	Operator: [Activates Lifepak 100 by removing its lid.]
00:00	Lifepak 100: "Connect electrodes."
00:30	Operator: [Completes connecting electrode paddles to patient's chest.]
00:30	Lifepak 100: "Is patient conscious?"
00:38	Operator: [Presses NO button.]
00:39	Lifepak 100: "Analyzing now. Do not touch patient!"

00:39	Lifepak 100: "Motion detected. Do not touch patient!" [This motion could be simply any movement of the patient's body, but the machine is warning the operator to sever all body-to-body contact with the patient, lest the operator be shocked also.]
00:40	Lifepak 100: "Analyzing now. Do not touch patient!"
00:41	Lifepak 100: "Motion detected. Do not touch patient!"
00:41	Lifepak 100: "Analyzing now. Do not touch patient!"
00:49	Lifepak 100: "Shock advised!"
00:51	Operator: [Presses SHOCK button.]
00:52	Lifepak 100: "Stand clear. Do not touch patient!"
01:01	Lifepak 100: [Delivers shock.]
01:02	Lifepak 100: "Do CPR, two breaths and fifteen chest compressions. Step completed?"
01:14	Operator: [Presses YES button.]
01:14	Lifepak 100: "Is patient conscious?"
01:20	Operator: [Presses NO button.]
01:21	Lifepak 100: "Analyzing now. Do not touch patient!"
01:23	Lifepak 100: "Motion detected. Do not touch patient!"
01:23	Lifepak 100: "Analyzing now. Do not touch patient!"
01:31	Lifepak 100: "No shock advised."
01:35	Lifepak 100: "Do CPR, two breaths and fifteen chest compressions. Step completed?"
01:42	[No response for sixty seconds.]

02:42   Lifepak 100: "Is patient conscious?"

02:43   Operator: [Presses YES button.]

LAST ENTRY

In less than three minutes, the patient was successfully defibrillated by the portable unit. Five minutes later, the rescue squad arrived and took the now alert and conscious arrhythmia victim to the hospital.

Initially, even cardiologists in the nonmainstream-electrophysiologist camp were concerned about how well devices like Lifepak 100 and Heart*Aid could detect ventricular fibrillation — and whether the units would advise a counter-shock when it was clinically not called for. But numerous studies have allayed these fears. In more than 95 percent of the cases analyzed, the portable defibrillators correctly identified ventricular fibrillation, without a glitch. And just as importantly, there have been no reports of aberrant shocks being delivered when fibrillation was not present.

It's difficult to resist the notion that prescribing portable defibrillators for all patients with severe arrhythmias, or potential arrhythmias due to coronary disease, could save thousands of lives each year. But the cost of these devices rules against it. Depending upon the final configuration, the Lifepak 100 runs $4,650 to $5,100; Heart*Aid, $4,700 to $9,000. Either of these units can be rented for $500 per month. At such prices portable defibrillators are simply too expensive for most patients. There are few arrhythmia patients like the one talked about in portable-defibrillator circles who bought three Lifepak 100s — one for his home, one for his office, and another for his boat — and hired trainers to teach all of those frequently near him, including his employees, how to use the unit. To him, money was of no concern; being able to live his life free from fear of sudden death was the only thing that mattered.

Unfortunately, physicians are hard pressed to find patients of such means; indeed, it is one of the sad ironies of being an arrhythmia victim that those who could profit most by owning a portable defibrillator are often already saddled by exorbitant medical expenses due to the catastrophic nature of their illnesses.

Third-party insurance coverage for the portable defibrillators is not a realistic option for those looking for financial help to buy or rent the devices. Insurance companies generally decide on a case-by-case basis whether to cover rentals, while Medicare takes a different tack: it offers no reimbursement at all for portable defibrillators. The federal government judges that these units are preventive medicine, not clinical treatments.

Says Boyd Kelly, deputy regional administrator of the federal Health Care Financing Administration: "Medicare only reimburses devices that are used for curing and healing, like home-dialysis machines."

It's difficult to see this position of Medicare as anything but illogical. Indeed, while the federal government grudgingly reimburses the implantable defibrillator — which does internally what the portable defibrillator does externally — and is known for its broad generosity across a discipline when it accepts the validity of a specific clinical strategy within a discipline, in this case it is unwilling to extend itself further and give appropriate and wider endorsement to a life-saving intervention.

Kelly adds: "We see the implantable defibrillator as a clinical treatment — and not preventative in nature — because it is only for patients who cannot be helped by surgery or medications."

Kelly turns away. He has the expression of a man who is trying to convince himself of the logic in his own position. He looks perplexed by how illogical it seems. After a long silence, he says with a shrug, "I know it's splitting hairs, but that's the basis for our position."

Recently there has been a new development in the portable defibrillator marketplace. Called MDphone, from Medphone Corporation (Paramus, New Jersey), this unit defibrillates a patient via communications lines, guided by a physician monitoring and supervising the rescue attempt at the local hospital.

On the patient side, MDphone consists of a ten-pound attaché case — the portable unit — with electrode paddles that attach to the victim's chest and wiring that plugs into the standard baseboard telephone jack. Via telecommunications this device "speaks" to the so-called control unit, located in the Coronary Care Unit or emergency room of a regional hospital. The control unit is essentially a personal computer with a CRT screen, a tape recorder, and a keyboard.

When a patient experiences symptoms of a heart disturbance, the patient or his or her partner dials the hospital automatically by opening up the attaché case. If the line to the control unit is busy, the call will be routed to a second hospital. When a connection is made with the control unit, the patient's medical chart is displayed on its CRT for the physician to study.

The physician now orally communicates with the patient unit, first advising how to put the paddles on the victim's chest in order to get an electrocardiogram readout on the computer screen. If the EKG indicates ventricular fibrillation or ventricular tachycardia, the control unit verifies adequate electrode contact with the patient's heart, sends out a signal to charge the patient unit, and then, with a keystroke, the physician can order MDphone to defibrillate. Obviously an ambulance is also dispatched to the patient's site simultaneously. With MDphone a nervous, panicking partner of a victim need only open the attaché case to automatically alert the rescue squad and also have the patient defibrillated.

On the other hand, of course, if no arrhythmia is noted in the electrocardiogram — indeed, if the patient is found to be suffering from indigestion or mild angina and not an arrhythmia attack — the physician at the control unit can suggest another course of action, such as medication, hospitalization, or a physician office visit.

To some electrophysiologists, MDphone is a desirable alternative to portable defibrillators like Lifepak 100 and Heart*Aid, because it ensures that a physician monitors and oversees the cardiac crisis from start to finish. Says Dr. Victor Parsonnet, clinical professor of surgery at the College of Medicine and Dentistry of New Jersey in Newark:

> It's more foolproof because a professional is involved throughout. First the physician makes a diagnosis over the telephone based on good, hard information: the patient's medical history and the current EKG. And if that diagnosis determines the need for defibrillation, then the physician himself fires the unit off. Other stock automatic defibrillators use a computer to read the vital signs and advise whether to discharge a countershock or not. The chances of computer errors and other mechanical foulups make these devices quite a bit more risky, I believe.

Perhaps so, but it is precisely the fact that human intervention from a remote site is required to defibrillate with MDphone that makes this unit a somewhat less acceptable security blanket for many patients than the other portable defibrillators. Two separate points of potential problems feed the perception that MDphone may not work when it must save a life.

First, at the time that the crisis phone call is made to the control unit, will it be manned with a physician already at the machine? Time wasted to call a physician to the control unit could mean the difference between life and death.

Second, because MDphone operates via telecommunications lines, what if the connection is spotty, the call doesn't go through, or the phone system is temporarily down? Medical emergencies — particularly arrhythmia attacks — are uncompromising in the face of mechanical glitches. Moreover, the fact that MDphone uses a telephone line as its umbilical cord means that it is a somewhat less than portable unit, but more a home or office defibrillator that can be permanently plugged into a dedicated phone jack.

To be fair, the manufacturer of MDphone is taking diligent steps to overcome any of these possible trouble spots. For one, it is working closely with participating hospitals to ensure proper staffing of the control unit. Further, it is developing a more failure-proof satellite-based dial-up system for the unit, so a clear connection can be gotten anywhere without plugging MDphone into a wall.

In one very important respect, though, MDphone has a clear leg up on other portable defibrillators — the purchase and use of it is reimbursed by third-party payers and Medicare. As the logic goes, the $5,000 patient unit and the additional $200 price tag it carries each time it is used is a companion to the $5,000 control unit that hospitals must buy; so MDphone is one component of a clinical treatment for heart disease and not a self-care "preventative" device like the other portable defibrillators.

Some cynics see the logic differently. To them, MDphone, like the implantable defibrillator, represents potentially significant financial returns to hospitals and clinicians; thus it would be difficult for the insurance carriers to rule against reimbursement.

Whichever portable defibrillator is taken home, one thing is certain: the lives of the patient and his or her family are changed irrevocably. Despite the numerous hours of training taken by all potential participants in out-of-hospital defibrillation, few are prepared for the mood swings from awkwardness to comfort, from fear to security, that accompany the presence of a portable defibrillator in their midst.

Peter G., a teenager from rural Stevensville, Virginia, whose father "died" from arrhythmias on the patient table of his cardiologist and was resuscitated, echoes the initial feelings of many in similar situations when he describes what it felt like at first to have a portable defibrillator sitting in his house: "It was always on my mind. It was kind of stressful to know that I may have to be the one to use it to save my dad's life. It scared me, really."

"That's a common first reaction, but it always changes before long," says Liane Chow, a specialist in cardiovascular nursing who trains portable defibrillator users. "After a while it becomes second nature to have the portable defibrillator around. It even becomes very comforting because the realization grows that for the first time they have a definite plan to cope with emergencies concerning their loved ones. What's most important is that soon they feel less hopeless in potentially frightening situations."

·13·

Scientists with MD Plates: The Keepers of the Future in Electrophysiology

P ERHAPS the most devastating fact about arrhythmias is that they operate silently and insidiously. Many of the 500,000 people who are felled each year in an irrevocable instant by cardiac arrest have shown no evidence of a problem before the pace of their hearts becomes frenzied and uncontrollable. To electrophysiologists it's a sad and uncompromising reality that the patients they are treating are those who have somehow survived their brushes with death; those they never get to care for simply fail to live through the grim battle.

Consequently, the next important clinical boundary that electrophysiologists must cross is to be able to predict an arrhythmia and identify those at immediate risk of dying from its fatal electrical design. Without that ability, electrophysiologists are relegated to the role of caretakers for the fortunate — for those lucky enough to be spit back by death; they're saddled with the frustration of being able to do nothing but mourn for those patients that got away. But if they could forecast the future performance of a heart — if they could accurately measure the inevitability of sudden cardiac arrest in any one person — these cardiologists would suddenly be in the privileged position of being able to defuse an otherwise imperceptible time bomb, one shrouded in the most carefully devised veils of secrecy.

For electrophysiologists, the effort to build a crystal ball that predicts the propensity for an individual's heart to be arrhythmic is a race against time, especially when one person dies from fibrillation or tachycardia each minute in the United States. But it's a race that is so exhilarating and potentially so rewarding that it has attracted a core group of the brightest "mixed-breed" physicians — those who are part clinician and part pure researcher — to its cause. These biologists, physicists, and computer scientists with MD plates are the keepers of the future in electrophysiology — interdisciplinarians who are dissecting and defining the very components of the mysterious diseased heart. Their mandate is complex but focused. Says Dr. Richard Cohen, the wunderkind director of the Harvard-Massachusetts Institute of Technology Center for Biomedical Engineering:

What we're looking for is the intrinsic property of the heart's hidden electrical substrata, that property that predisposes a person to spontaneous arrhythmias. There are some individuals who are electrically unstable and have a higher probability of spontaneous arrhythmias — that we know, although we can't identify these individuals yet. So we're trying to determine the underlying cardiac instability among these people. Our goal is to develop a technique to detect latent electrical instability.

By combining raw clinical and arithmetic data with the theories of cardiology and the axioms of the life sciences, researchers like Cohen are building detailed and precise models of the heart and its properties on computers. From the edge of the pulse beat through the wavelike electric current that suffuses the heart, these graphic cardiac replicas first emulate the smooth motion of the normal sinus rhythm. Then, when a jagged cadence is introduced, the image on the computer screen shivers and shakes in frenzied fibrillation.

The work of these investigators is without precedent and is dependent on a new scientific method that runs counter to the two prevailing and established poles of cardiac research, represented by those who, on the one hand, see the heart as a black box and, on the other hand, by those to whom cardiac details are their sustenance.

The "black box theorists" view the heart as an organ that is indecipherable when examined in its component parts. Any knowledge of cardiac activities, according to these broad-view researchers, is obtained by taking a holistic snapshot of the cardiac muscle and not by analyzing its operations at a micro level.

The "cardiac detail seekers" counter that the heart is made up of an infinite number of elements, and unless each element is marked, measured, and defined, the hidden truths of the cardiac muscle will remain inscrutably out of reach.

Neither approach is correct, say Cohen and his colleagues at universities around the country, when it comes to understanding tachycardia and fibrillation. Tachycardia and fibrillation occur on a local, regionalized level so the black-box notion will only generate platitudes and generalizations without substance: it is akin to trying to identify the chemical makeup of lunar rocks using only a telescope, that is, without obtaining samples for hands-on examination.

And as for component-by-component research of the heart, scientifically it is seductive. Practically, though, it only leads to overanalysis and an exaggerated enthusiasm for "discoveries" that are curious but at the same time a diversion from the real aim, which is to understand arrhythmias. Says Arthur Winfree, theoretical biologist at the University of Arizona and one of the leading arrhythmia hunters of the 1980s:

> The tendency of many scientists is to amass data and then find some way to fit all of it into the research — that

is, to use all the knowledge we've gathered to make the most painstakingly realistic model of what is being investigated. That sounds like a cogent approach, but it's fraught with failure. The fact is you get hopelessly lost in the forest of detail and end up more confused than when you started.

To understand arrhythmias it makes far more sense to try to select a few details that you imagine are the most crucial details — and that's where sound scientific judgment comes in — and make a caricature of the heart. This caricature — actually an oversimplified model with some detail — as it turns out, does show us fundamental things. This approach works primarily because fibrillation is a disorder of the organization of the heartbeat rather than a malfunction of macro elements of the heart, such as the individual cardiac fibers. It affects the timing of activity in the heart fibers in respect to one another, but it does not necessarily affect the heart fibers themselves.

Winfree came to the study of cardiac rhythms from his research in the early 1980s on another natural system that is as precise and ordered as the heartbeat: circadian clocks, the intrinsic twenty-four-hour cycles most organisms possess. Winfree found that a single brief stimulus, if it was properly timed during the "vulnerable phase," could cause organisms that were extremely rhythmic to lose their regular rhythms. At about the same time of this discovery, on two separate occasions, colleagues died of sudden cardiac arrest in Winfree's presence.

"I was a helpless witness," he says.

Goaded by the horror of these deaths, Winfree began to investigate cardiac rhythms. He posited that maybe the heart also had vulnerable periods when a single aberrant impulse could send the heartbeat into disarray. Perhaps, he thought, it is the refractory period during which cells are resting and not contracting, a time when under normal conditions cardiac cells are unable to accept electrical stimuli.

In a massive effort, Winfree constructed a series of complex mathematical and geometrical formulas which, he said, proved that if the timing is just right an entire heart can become arrhythmic when an ectopic or abnormal beat is introduced at localized, regional sites. Using the perfect symmetry of how numbers react to each other under given conditions and applying it to knowledge about the heart gleaned by cardiologists, Winfree produced what he felt was an indisputable view of the cardiac electrical conduction processes. This was unique and exciting research. It was the first true abstract model of the heart based on real cardiac properties.

Still, few in the cardiology community knew quite what to make of Winfree's work. On one level, some thought, it offered nothing new. It was merely a model that mathematically and graphically depicted the mechanics of what occurs daily at electrophysiology labs across the country when damaged hearts are stimulated by an electrical impulse to set off an incipient arrhythmia so that it can be analyzed and treated.

On another level, though, this was an invitation to investigate chaos. As Winfree applied his mathematical formulas to hearts of different physical characteristics, vastly varying arrhythmias occurred. From one heart to another the patterns of arrhythmia produced by the models seemed entirely random and disorderly. Though there was an internal organization to the disarray in each individual heart, there was no general pattern that obtained among all hearts. Using Winfree's model to write an equation that would identify all individuals with potentially arrhythmic hearts and the kind of arrthymias they might exhibit seemed an utterly impossible task.

One researcher found this out the hard way. Studying balls of cells from the hearts of chicken embryos, Dr. Leon Glass at McGill University in Montreal discovered that when an artificial electrical stimulus was applied to these cells a variety of cardiac rhythms resulted. For instance, in one arrhythmic heart the number of healthy beats between the abnormal ones always came from a sequence of odd numbers — 1, 3, or 5. But in a second arrhythmic chicken embryo heart, the number of normal beats that alternated with the ectopic ones were derived from a vastly different numerical pattern — 2, 3, 8, 11, 14 . . .

Says Glass: "The dynamics of these arrhythmic rhythms are much richer than anybody would have guessed. They're entirely chaotic."

Chaotic, indeed. Still, chaos need not be disorderly, reasoned Richard Cohen at the Harvard-Massachusetts Institute of Technology Center for Biomedical Engineering, who took Winfree's and Glass's conclusions one giant step further. Perhaps chaos is unruly. But without organization? No.

Cohen, the thirty-seven-year-old whiz kid of advanced arrhythmia research, began as a physics and chemistry major at Harvard and then got an M.D. and Ph.D. in physics through a cooperative program between Harvard and M.I.T. He borrowed his notion of orderly chaos from the landmark research of an M.I.T. colleague, Mitchell Feigenbaum, who stunned the physics and science communities in the early 1980s with a theory that debunks the idea of chaos being governed entirely by chance. According to Feigenbaum, even if it is difficult to discern, in life as in nature there are remarkably elegant patterns underlying the transition from order to disorder.

Feigenbaum has termed his concept the chaos theory. Its central point is that chaos is everywhere. You can see it in the way that cigarette smoke rising evenly suddenly breaks into a swirling spiral or in the way that a faucet drips at first steadily and then, without warning, randomly. But there are a limited number of mathematical and physiological paths that nature has for the movement from order to disorder.

The idea is that small shifts in what precipitates an event quickly become overwhelming differences in the outcome of the event. Feigenbaum describes this by the rugged phrase, "sensitive dependence on initial conditions." Put more elegantly, it is best expressed by the metaphor that the movement of a butterfly's wings as it departs a flower in Peking affects the weather a month later in New York City. By understanding initial conditions occuring during a period of order, what will happen in the subsequent period of disorder or chaos can be better understood and anticipated.

To Cohen, Feigenbaum's chaos theory was eye-opening. It

meant that rather than looking at the end result — that is the types of normal and abnormal heartbeats that made up an arrhythmia, as Winfree and Glass were doing — it would be wiser to investigate the precipitators — the initial conditions — of the arrhythmia.

To prove that the chaos theory is applicable to cardiology, Cohen first produced models of healthy cardiac conduction on massive Digital Equipment Corporation "VAX" computers with sophisticated graphic capabilities. He took a normal human heart, sectioned it, made a Kodachrome transparency of each section, and finally digitized the Kodachromes to create a three-dimensional representation of the heart. Then, he added cardiac physiological data in the form of algorithms and equations that made the computerized heart come to life.

To examine the onset of arrhythmia, in an initial experiment, Cohen changed the data parameters so that the computerized cardiac system was less stable and was prone to spontaneous fibrillation.

He was shocked by the pattern he found each time he compromised the stability of his model. He had uncovered a quirk — a precursor as much as a precipitator — that seemed to indicate that an arrhythmia is about to occur.

We began to see a type of electrical alternation that consistently preceded arrhythmia. That is, one heart beat would be of one shape and the next beat took on an entirely different shape. It was an A-B-A-B-A-B-A-B type of pattern. In our computer simulations this electrical alternans [alternation] always preceded the onset of any type of heart rhythm disturbance, particularly fibrillation.

Cohen tried his discovery out on dogs. He cooled the animal's heart down, which makes it vulnerable and susceptible to arrhythmias, and then monitored the heartbeat, looking for his precipitator to chaos.

The same thing occurred. Each time the same A-B-A-B electrical alternation occurred in the dog's heartbeat just before it became arrhythmic, as we first saw on our computer model.

Just a clue, but a potentially important one. This was the first hint that the body tips off the impending arrival of an arrhythmic event through a subtle variation in the heart beat.

Subsequent to his discovery of electrical alternation, using his computerized models, Cohen came up with yet another extremely significant cardiac intimation of chaos, one tied directly to the most intricate electrical nuances of the heart.

The cardiac electrical cycle has two phases. There's the highly synchronous depolarization phase, when the cells are refractory or unable to accept an electrical stimulus. They're simply insensitive to the electrical activity around them. During the shift to refractoriness, one heart region becomes depolarized, which causes a neighboring group of cells to depolarize and so on down the line. Depolarization spreads through the cardiac muscle like a wave retreating over the sand back toward the ocean. A region remains depolarized for a set period of time — that is, until its local biological clock tells it that the rest period is up.

Then there's the asynchronous repolarization phase when the cells are recharged. Because each cardiac region has a separate timer attached to it, repolarization is not a propagating current, but rather a patchy event. Some regions are repolarized, while other regions remain refractory for another moment or two. In short, during any one instant, different cells of the heart are switched on, while others are switched off, even though all of the cells were depolarized in a relatively synchronous fashion.

Considering this sensitive electrical conduction structure in the heart, with finely tuned on and off switches operating in patterns of remarkable organization and synchrony, Cohen wondered whether slight shifts in the depolarization and re-polarization phases could be trigger points to fibrillation.

What happens if a new wave of depolarization impinges upon a region of tissue, some areas of which are still refractory and some areas of which are not?

Running this well-established experimental scenario through his computer model of the heart, Cohen discovered that the new incoming wave of depolarization fractionates because it is forced to go around the already refractory islands of tissue. This splintering of incoming depolarization signals leaves behind loops of skewed electrical activity in which already-repolarized regions are shut down prematurely by the new wave and depolarized regions are unable to repolarize. Like switches short-circuiting, cells in the heart blink on and off without resonance and pattern.

We incorporated this dispersion of refractoriness idea over a scale on the order of millimeters. We'e not talking about from one cell to another. It actually occurs over a microscopic spatial region.

Cohen calls this phenomenon period doubling after Mitchell Feigenbaum's notion that in a natural system it is a cascade of period doublings — disorderly events that build upon each other to create still more disorder — that finally result in a chaotic state. For electrophysiology, this is significant because it suggests that new aberrant instructions to shut down the internal circuitry, impinging on the normal, healthy instructions, can grow more insidious and omnipotent as they travel through the cardiac cells and can ultimately be the key that throws the heart's rhythms into disarray.

Cohen's research is very new and, unfortunately, still years away from practical clinical applications. But it defines a hope-ful direction. It clearly proves that if his computer models are a faithful replica of the heart, then there are detectable signals — perhaps many triggers — that foreshadow the imminence of an arrhythmia.

Detectable, of course, in this case is an extremely relative term. Says Cohen:

It would take a microprocessor or minicomputer-based instrument to analyze one or more surface leads of an ECG [EKG] and the fine details of the structure of the electrocardiographic complexes of the heart in order to detect in a real heart any of the subtle variabilities that we're finding on our computerized models. The human eye is not designed to look at the heart's electrical properties and identify subtle changes and, of course, the human observer only has the patience and the discipline to examine 2, 3, or 4 heart beats, not several hundred. A computer, on the other hand, can analyze hundreds of heartbeats rapidly by using statistical methods.

But the importance of this research is that we obviously can't do invasive testing on a large population. So eventually, with the help of a computer, we will hopefully be able to noninvasively screen people at risk, suggest follow-up diagnostic procedures and help guide treatment strategies. I want to emphasize, we're very far away from doing that. This is a long-term goal. What we're focusing on now is simply trying to understand the mechanisms of conduction abnormalities.

Not all of the interdisciplinarians trying to define the nature of arrhythmias are content with using computer models of the heart. The argument against these models, as expressed by one leading electrophysiologist, goes this way:

Computer cardiac models are nothing but artificial depictions of reality and potentially the source of dangerous misinformation. Though they may be mathematically cogent representations of the heart, they are not true and animate physiological artifacts — thus, they are of dubious clinical merit.

To counter the imperfections of computer models, some researchers are experimenting with recording the performance of the heart's electrical system using dozens of electrodes impaled at once on the surface of real hearts. Data gathered directly from the beating heart through these electrodes are analyzed and organized by a computer that drafts a road map of the heart being studied, showing its distinct and discrete electrical activities.

The computer graphics produced from the electrical activity of a live beating heart are of such immense detail and substance that one glance at them makes tangible and comprehensible the somewhat abstract notion of what an arrhythmia actually "looks" like. On the computer monitor, semicircular dot-matrix pulses emerge from a dead-center heartbeat, resembling ripples in a pond emanating from a dropped rock or signals coming out of a radio tower in the line drawings of the 1930s. A healthy heart rhythm is depicted by free-flowing waves that move in and recede in organized cycles; but an arrhythmia is portrayed as closely-bound, thick lines, moving in a disorganized sequence across the surface of the heart.

Of course, creating a heart map is all in a day's work for clinical electrophysiologists at the leading arrhythmia centers who commonly snake between one and four electrode catheters through a patient's heart, trying to induce an arrhythmia and discern its so-called activation sequence — that is, a blueprint of where the arrhythmia begins and the path it travels through the heart. But while this electrode catheter technique is satisfactory as a diagnostic tool for electrophysiology lab procedures, it is entirely unsatisfactory for research purposes. It leads to no clear understanding of the source of arrhythmias and how they function.

Says Dr. Raymond Ideker, a cardiac pathologist at the Duke University Medical Center:

Arrhythmias are often initiated by several different cycles in the heart. Frequently, multiple arrhythmia activation fronts coexist in the heart simultaneously. In each of these instances it is critical that data from all cardiac measuring points be acquired at the same time.

To hear Ideker talk is a curious experience. A computerphile in M.D.'s clothing, Ideker is as at home discussing multiple-chip arrays as he is discussing anomalies of the ventricles. He's a high-tech Mr. Wizard who says he realized long ago that scientists don't save lives, but only hand physicians the weapons to go to war with death. Still, doctors are the ones fighting the battle.

After I graduated from college in 1968, I went to work for IBM as a systems analyst. I had never seen a computer before I went to work for them. I also didn't know exactly what I wanted to do professionally at that point. I enjoyed working with computers but after about a year I came to the conclusion that I wanted to do something practical with my life — I wanted it to have some greater meaning. So I went to medical school at the University of Tennessee where, besides my M.D., I got a degree in physiology. In doing that I combined my interest in electronics with clinical work — and I became involved in electrophysiology. With my rounded science background I discovered that there are so many important things that I could work on. So I decided to pick an area that affects the lives of people. I made it my long-term goal to use what I knew about computers, physiology, and medicine to understand fibrillation and learn how to prevent it.

To take recordings of the beating heart from multiple electrodes, Ideker and his colleagues at Duke, particularly Dr. William Smith, devised a cloth mesh sock — it looks like a hair net — with electrodes embedded in it. When maps are to be drawn of the ventricular electrical activation sequence the sock is slipped over the bottom half of the heart and anchored at its base with sutures. Once the sock is tightly attached to the heart, the electrodes make contact with the cardiac surface. The latest version of Ideker's multiple-electrode cardiac monitor has 128 separate electrodes or contact points.

Gathering of data from the sock is controlled by a microprocessor, which filters the incoming information (blocking out extraneous heart "noise") and converts the analog signals entering the electrodes into streams of digital bits and bytes that the computer can interpret. By pointing a so-called light pen at choices on the computer screen or on maps appearing sequentially on the monitor, a physican can start data acquisition, select a heart beat that he wants to see in more detail, and obtain a heart map in less than a minute.

Currently most of Ideker's maps are generated from canine hearts — which are purposely tampered with and made arrhythmic — though he is making recordings from some human hearts during open heart operations.

"As long as we're in there doing surgery on a patient's heart, we're also going to do some research," he says.

Ideker is a humanist and not entirely comfortable with killing dogs to record abnormal electrical conduction in their hearts, but he is convinced that there is no other way. While it hurts Ideker to be a target of the argument against animal studies, in his mind the good of what he does far outweighs the perceived evil.

Animal studies are necessary in our case, plain and simple. We cannot do all of this by computer simulation. I wish we could. I hate it that we have to kill animals. But my rationale is that the animals are going to be killed by the pound anyway. Fortunately, in our studies we don't require conscious animals and it's not the kind of horror stuff that the animal groups show in pictures. Here's a case where animal studies are preventing something really bad from being done on people.

Still, in an almost eerie afterthought, Ideker adds that animal studies are not in this case, or any case, a truly desirable replacement for human experimentation.

We've done enough mapping with humans to give me more than a little concern that under too many circumstances the heart of a dog reacts far differently than that of a person.

So far Ideker's heart maps have yielded little useful information about how fibrillation occurs and what foreshadows it, but they depict with uncanny detail the face of an arrhythmia and the territory it travels. This, according to Ideker, is priceless data. "Knowing what your enemy looks like is the key to knowing how your enemy thinks," he says

Ideker is convinced that his approach, far better than computer modeling, holds the key to the secrets of arrhythmias. In describing his aims, though, Ideker echoes the desperation of so many in the electrophysiology community, who understand that their inability to forecast and short-circuit that next sudden death from arrhythmia makes the splash of their impressive post–cardiac arrest clinical achievements pale into a frustrating fizzle.

The hope is that soon we will be able to take people and identify those who at first blush appear to be at ten percent risk of sudden cardiac arrest from arrhythmia, and then with deeper analysis divide them into those at an actual thirty percent risk and those at an actual two percent risk. At this point this seems like an impossible goal, but I have to go on the idea that the more information we can gather and the more we can learn, the more likely we are to come up with some useful way to predict who is at risk — to create the list of who is likely to die soon from this devious condition.

·14·

The Answer

Aⁱ sk anyone who knows him and they will tell you that Dr. Michel Mirowski, the director of the Coronary Care Unit at Baltimore's Sinai Hospital, is an extremely humble man. Never mind the lurking suspicion that Mirowski uses deference and humility as a lasso to ensnare you deeper in conversation, in order to convert you to his cause; he is still a man of modesty. An Eastern European Jew who, in his youth, successfully dodged Hitler's storm troopers, Mirowski uses verbal nuance and the twinkling of an old man's eye to make sure he's heard and listened to. Thus, because it's so uncharacteristic of him, it's difficult not to take notice when taking a direct, unwavering stance, Mirowski proclaims that his invention — this little black box that he's holding in his hand, the one with crooked catheters dangling crudely from its chassis — is nothing less than the key to life for arrhythmia victims.

It represents not only a reduction but virtually an eradication of sudden death by arrhythmia.

Mirowski's device is a marvel of miniaturized electronics that carries a bulky appellation: automatic implantable cardioverter defibrillator, or AICD. Mirowski is not the only one to sing its praises; it has electrophysiologists buzzing with plaudits and excitement as well. Jeremy Ruskin, for one, is effusive in his support for the AICD.

> The implantable defibrillator is revolutionizing cardiology. It is one of a small number of developments that this generation will get to see which will clearly change the course of the way that we practice medicine. It's the single most important advance to date in the treatment of life-threatening ventricular arrhythmias.

A glance at the short history of the AICD shows that the hyperbole surrounding it is not without foundation. Indications are that this device is the closest thing to The Answer that clinicians in all disciplines look for — it's the Miracle Vaccine; it's the Heralded Solution. For electrophysiologists, it's the counterpoint to risky and dangerous drug therapies for arrhythmias.

Weighing a little more than one-half pound and distinctly smaller than a paperback book, the pulse generator portion of the implantable defibrillator is tucked beneath the skin in the abdominal region of a patient, while two of its electrodes are sutured to the ventricles of the heart. When the patient develops ventricular tachycardia or fibrillation, the AICD detects the rapid rhythm and delivers a very brief shock intended to restore the heart to its normal rhythm. In most instances, this initial shock will end the arrhythmia. If it doesn't, the implantable defibrillator recycles itself and prepares to output as many as three additional shocks of higher electrical energy until the tachycardia or fibrillation is stilled.

Since late 1985, when the Food and Drug Administration approved the AICD for general use among arrhythmia victims, well over 4,000 of the devices have been implanted in patients worldwide (as of June 1988). The statistics of success are uniformly remarkable.

In studies conducted at numerous sites from Stanford University Medical Center in California to Massachusetts General Hospital, the one-year arrhythmia mortality rate for those with AICDs installed is always under 2 percent, usually closer to 1.5 percent. This same group of critically ill patients, when treated with the methods of traditional cardiology, has a mortality rate of approximately 30 percent.

Looked at from yet another viewpoint, what makes the survival rate among AICD implantees most significant is that currently only the so-called "last resort" patients — that is, only those patients in which all other clinical alternatives have been attempted and failed — are candidates for the implantable defibrillator. The AICD is not offering life to those who could find it some other way; it is literally reclaiming the statistically dead.

One of these statistics was James P., a fifty-five-year-old Cleveland lawyer who had a ten-year history of coronary artery disease and concomitant arrhythmias when he arrived at the Cleveland Clinic in August 1981. At the time, electrophysiology techniques such as resection and freezing the electrically damaged area through cryosurgery were still not perfected, so pharmacological solutions were all that James P.'s physicians had at their disposal.

Unfortunately for James P., as for so many other patients, drugs simply did not silence his arrhythmia. Despite trials with numerous drugs, the arrhythmia was easily reinduced in the electrophysiology lab when James P.'s heart was stimulated; each drug was simply ineffective. So with no other alternatives, James P.'s physicians sent him back into the real world, his arrhythmia as dangerous and threatening as ever.

"Our expectations were that he wouldn't survive through the end of the year," says one of James P.'s cardiologists, at the time a resident at the Cleveland Clinic.

As it turns out, James P. surprised his doctors. He lived to see New Year's Eve, though barely. Even the simplest of activities — walking to the kitchen from his living room or going outside to get the mail — were efforts of such magnitude that they became as difficult to perform as running a marathon would be for most healthy people.

Then, in March 1982, while sitting in his living room watching television, James P.'s heart suddenly started contracting in random rhythms like static from a radio and his body twitched three or four times. The very next moment, he collapsed.

Fortunately, he was revived by paramedics called by his wife, and James P. was once again at the Cleveland Clinic. His physicians felt that their backs were completely against the wall with this case. So they made a bold move for that period in medical history. Emulating the just-discovered technique that was then making the rounds of the electrophysiology community, James P.'s physicians decided to try to excise the region of the heart responsible for the arrhythmia.

However, during investigations with catheter electrodes to locate the earliest activation site of the arrhythmia, a new roadblock was thrown in the doctors' way. James P.'s arrhythmia was sited deep in the inner walls of his heart, an area with which his physicians could not confidently tamper without risking irrevocable damage to the cardiac muscle.

"He may have been on his last legs, but at least he was alive," says the Cleveland Clinic resident. "Maybe we should've attempted excision, but we simply did not feel like we'd be successful. Also, during this period of investigation, we found that a combination of the drugs Amiodarone and propranolol partially controlled his ventricular tachycardia, so we decided to send him back out with those prescriptions."

For a while the drugs did work — but only for a short period. During the next year most of James P.'s arrhythmia symptoms subsided and his quality of life actually improved to the point where simple activities were no longer daunting. But after a year, by late 1983, the breathlessness returned — this time even when James P. was just lying down. He had developed pulmonary toxicity to Amiodarone, an all-too-common side effect of the drug. His lungs were reacting unfavorably to the

Amiodarone and James P. was at risk for extensive pulmonary damage. The drug was discontinued and, once again, James P.'s arrhythmia returned.

At the Cleveland Clinic, James P. was put through yet another round of drug testing. All conventional and investigational pharmacological options were tried and retried. None worked. James P. was once again released from the hospital and recurrent, life-threatening ventricular tachycardia became a monthly fact of life for him.

James P.'s physicians were now grasping for any solution to his disease, as it grew progressively more severe each day. At first, they had written James P. off as another mortality statistic. But after three years of hopes and then disappointments with this patient — and after three years of witnessing his valiant struggle to live — they had an emotionally vested commitment to his survival. So after analyzing the details of the case — his arrhythmia had worsened steadily over thirty-six months; all traditionally known options were exhausted; the patient was at the stage of last resort — James P.'s doctors concluded that his only chance for a return to a normal quality of life and, indeed, survival was the implantable defibrillator.

This was an extremely courageous decision. Though the federal Food and Drug Administration did not approve the AICD for general use until nearly 1986, the device had been implanted in humans since 1980 in carefully controlled experimental clinical trials. It was at the same stage of the regulatory process — that is, not yet allowed for widespread use — that the artificial heart is today. So in recommending implantation of the AICD, James P.'s physicians were calling for nothing less than pure experimentation. The risks were enormous, but the gamble was the last clinical card that they held.

Ready to try anything to survive, James P. immediately agreed with his doctors' assessment of his case, and on May 7, 1984, he was wheeled into the Cleveland Clinic electrophysiology lab for the initial stage of AICD implantation. While the patient was still awake, the first of the implantable defibrillator's electrode catheters was inserted into his subclavian vein — on his left side — and, following the trail of bloodlines, it was positioned at the junction of the superior vena cava and the right atrium. Insertion of another AICD catheter electrode followed. This one was positioned in James P.'s right ventricle. James P. was taken back to the CCU ward where he spent a restless night.

The next day James P. was brought to the operating room. This time he was given general anesthesia and slept through the most dangerous part of the implantation procedure. A horizontal incision was made across the left side of his chest, the heart was exposed, and the third AICD electrode was sutured on to the patient's left ventricle. Finally, the implantable defibrillator itself was tucked neatly under the skin in the paraumbilical region of his abdomen, right next to his navel. The AICD was wired, charged, and ready to operate.

The postoperative period was quiet, and four days later James P. was wheeled into the electrophysiology lab for testing of the implantable defibrillator. Paddles were attached to his chest. A stimulating current was sent into James P.'s heart and its steady rhythms dissipated into uncontrolled tachycardia. The AICD waited 13 seconds, vigilantly ticking off the moments until it was evident that this arrhythmia was not just a transient event. Finally, the implantable defibrillator delivered a 27-joule shock through its electrodes and then paused to assess whether the tachycardia had been halted.

"The shock was uncomfortable because it was unexpected," says James P. "I didn't even know I was in arrhythmia and here comes this sudden inside-out punch in my chest. It was painful; I won't deny that. But it was tolerable."

There was no need to deliver a second shock. The arrhythmia disappeared. The AICD had performed perfectly. The next day James P. was discharged from the Cleveland Clinic. Gone were the drug-induced fatigue and lethargy that shadowed him as he awaited his next cardiac arrest. Though he was still somewhat tentative about plunging headlong back into the normal activities of life, it was now a psychological barrier that he had to cross and not a physiological barrier.

Six weeks later, though he really wasn't aware of it, James P. suffered his first posthospital tachycardia. What he was aware of, though, was how the implantable defibrillator reacted to it. The AICD's arrhythmia reversion shock was again sharp and disconcerting. For a split second James P.'s chest jolted forward, as if he had been punched at full force in his back. But seconds later his body relaxed. And his heart beat returned to a stable rhythm.

James P. still suffers an arrhythmic event monthly, but because of the programmed reaction of the AICD, he never even feels his heart rhythms failing. What's more, his life is not statistically in danger any longer.

Since James P. received his implantable defibrillator, much has changed. For one, no longer is the AICD an experimental device. Indeed, now the only reason why more are not installed in arrhythmia patients is that the manufacturer simply cannot produce them quickly enough to keep up with demand.

The AICD is accepted by electrophysiologists as the ticket to renewed life for many of their patients — as the means to offer their patients a permanent chance to step cleanly away from the vicious cycle that arrhythmias represent. But as in much of the history of electrophysiological advances, the development of the implantable defibrillator met with sturdy resistance from the traditionalist, conservative health care community. The story of how the AICD was conceived and built offers a unique look at how persistence can overcome roadblocks and surmount the opprobrium of those opposed to scientific change among the nation's medical establishment.

If there was one seminal moment that was the inspiration for the implantable defibrillator, it was the day in 1967 when Dr. Julian A., one of Michel Mirowski's closest friends and a leading physician in Israel, collapsed suddenly from severe tachycardia. Mirowski, who was then chief of cardiology at the Israeli hospital Asaf Haroseh, saw clearly that his friend was dying. Drugs were prescribed, but they did little to thwart Julian A.'s arrhythmia.

Mirowski felt depressed. A general dull funk settled on him, but he couldn't quite pinpoint the cause of his malaise. He knew it wasn't only that Julian A. was ill. There was more to it than that.

A few days later, Mirowski was having tea with his wife. He sat quietly, brooding. Concerned, she asked him, "What's the problem, Michel? Why are you so worried all the time?"

Without thinking, he blurted out: "Julian's going to drop dead one day very soon and there's nothing that I can do about it. With all my medical training in cardiology, I am completely unable to save his life; it is hanging by a thread."

Two weeks later, while dining, Julian A. collapsed and died, a victim of cardiac arrest from arrhythmia. But except for sadness over the loss of his friend, Mirowski barely flinched emotionally. He had already made peace with the inevitability of Julian A.'s death and with what his response to it should be. As it turns out, in the clarity of that moment fourteen days earlier with his wife at tea, Mirowski's depression had lifted. In that instant, activism replaced pessimism.

Mirowski is direct about the meaning of Julian A.'s death: it was a blessing. It catalyzed Mirowski's resolve to build a device that could save future patients from dying suddenly because of arrhythmias. That such a device was needed became undeniable when Mirowski considered the extreme impracticability of the two methods by which his friend could have been kept alive: first, he could have been kept permanently in the hospital's Coronary Care Unit, where external defibrillators are available — the kind used to countershock and defuse purposely induced arrhythmias in the electrophysiology lab.

Notes Mirowski: "That solution was not feasible, because otherwise Julian A. was quite active and healthy. It would be committing him to life imprisonment to put Julian A. in a CCU ward where he could be tethered to the defibrillator as if it was an umbilical cord."

The second method for keeping Julian A. from death was even more ludicrous: hire a physician with an external defibrillator in tow to walk behind Julian A. around the clock. Should Julian A.'s heart rhythms fail, the doctor could revive him and reestablish a normal pulse beat with the defibrillator.

Faced with such unacceptable medical strategies for an illness like heart arrhythmias, which when untreated offers nothing but imminent death, Mirowski decided to develop a feasible response that obviated the traditional limitations of out-of-hospital resuscitation schemes.

> It occurred to me that there was only one solution: build an implantable device that could do what we're doing in the coronary care unit — that is, that could monitor the patient's heart continuously, promptly identify the onset of malignant arrhythmias, and then deliver the antidote. Moreover, these functions must be performed automatically so the high-risk patient is protected from the consequences of arrhythmia whenever and wherever he is stricken by it.
>
> So with this solution as my goal, I took out a sheet of paper and wrote down my design considerations. As I saw it the device must: 1) perform long-term monitoring; 2) detect arrhythmias reliably; 3) deliver a countershock effectively; 4) be small enough for implantation in the body; and 5) be built of suitable materials so that it is compatible with the body's chemistry.

For the better part of the next year, Mirowski honed and fine-tuned on paper the design for his implantable defibrillator. He knew that in late 1968 he would be moving to the United States to become director of the Coronary Care Unit at Sinai in Baltimore, and his plan was to get a series of grants and then build the AICD as a research project at the hospital. But soon after he arrived in this country, his carefully constructed timetable was altered when it became clear that Mirowski would have a difficult time obtaining money from a granting agency to build the implantable defibrillator. The mainstream medical community was simply not comfortable with his plans to design the device. Electrophysiology itself was considered a renegade discipline trampling on traditional cardiological notions, and the thought that equipment was being developed to spur electrophysiology was galling to the conservative powers-that-be in health care.

But even without the help of the National Institutes of Health — the prime supporter of basic medical research in the U.S. with its high-nine-figure annual research treasure chest — and the National Science Foundation, Mirowski was undaunted. He teamed up with a Sinai colleague, Dr. Morton Mower, and the two men began building the implantable defibrillator on their own time, relying entirely on their own money. Setting up shop in the basement of Sinai, next to the animal laboratory, Mirowski and Mower spent virtually every waking hour that they weren't scheduled to work in the hospital's wards piecing together the conceptual and developmental riddles of the AICD.

> We kept our costs down by using our imagination. A dog for clinical research could cost a hundred and fifty dollars under normal circumstances in those days. But not having the luxury of buying too many dogs at those prices, we started purchasing the animals from the pound for one dollar apiece. Then we bought electronic parts from discount catalogs or used extra components that were destined for the trash bin at Sinai's Bio-Electrical Engineering Laboratory. And without federal funding we were freed from the costs of maintaining fellowships and writing progress reports.

As word traveled throughout the cardiology community that Mirowski's attempt to design an AICD was continuing apace, the backstage campaign against the implantable defibrillator went public and escalated into open hostility.

In 1972, with Mirowski and Mower making plodding but consistent progress on the AICD — two years earlier, for example, the first experimental implantable defibrillator had been successfully tested on dogs — the medical journal *Circulation,* the official publication of the American Heart Association, ran a three-page editorial panning the device and calling for the development effort to cease. This editorial opened Mirowski's eyes wide.

> Our attempts to build an implantable defibrillator definitely touched some nerves.

Indeed it did; for there is no other explanation for the kinds of specious and dubious arguments that were raised against the implantable defibrillator in the *Circulation* editorial:

> . . . That the heart will be injured [by the use of the implantable defibrillator] is certain; the only uncertainty is its extent. . . .
>
> If the patient with such an implanted device is found dead, numerous questions will loom, including the gnawing doubt that electrocution [from the implantable defibrillator] may have been a factor. . . .
>
> The promulgators of . . . [the implantable defibrillator] have stated: "It is too early to determine exactly the indications and contraindications of the . . . [implantable] defibrillator." Should not such a question be answered before social energies are expended? If no indications can be clearly defined, why dissipate scarce health resources? . . .
>
> There is no evidence that the individual who has a single bout of ventricular fibrillation is likely to have recurrences. . . . [T]he implanted defibrillator system represents an imperfect solution in search of a plausible and practical application. . . .

There are two quiet, but telling ironies lurking in the backdrop of this editorial that are impossible to see from the face of it.

First, this piece in *Circulation* was based on research funded by the NIH, which was apparently willing to provide money to lambast the implantable defibrillator in print but was entirely unwilling at the time to pay for any of the development costs for the device. This despite the fact that the NIH is usually not a very discriminating agency about what it funds. It regularly proffers large sums of money to many research efforts of questionable and nonlifesaving value, such as projects that study hormonal development in butterflies.

Second, the editorial was written in part by Dr. Bernard Lown, who, as discussed in chapter 3, just ten years earlier had led a landmark in-hospital defibrillation of a patient's nearly fatal arrhythmia after anti-arrhythmic drugs utterly failed to slow its pace. This procedure, performed by Lown and his colleagues at Peter Bent Brigham Hospital in Boston, was one of the first clinical showpieces of electrophysiology and highlighted the significant fact that an arrhythmic human heart reverts to a normal rhythm when countershocked or defibrillated. At the time, Lown commented with passion about the all too common deleterious effects of anti-arrhythmic drug strategies and about how efficacious synchronized countershock was for reverting an arrhythmia.

Then, Lown was speaking as a member of the cardiac avant-garde — as an electrophysiologist. Subsequently, though, Lown had seemingly become out of step with breakthroughs in arrhythymia research. Thus, in 1972 he was writing as an apologist for the traditionalists, citing as effective strategies for arrhythmia patients such failed and expensive approaches as long-term stays in the coronary care units; "surgical correction" — bypasses and arterial grafts, the mainstays of old-line cardiologists; and, against his own first-hand knowledge, drug therapies.

And beyond the ironies of Lown's apparent revisionism, there are also questionable medical statements, which Lown presents as fact, that make the *Circulation* editorial so surprising. With Lown's background in electrophysiology it is difficult to understand how he arrived at conclusions such as:

That the heart will be injured [by the use of the implantable defibrillator] is certain; the only uncertainty is its extent. . . .[and] There is no evidence that the individual who has a single bout of ventricular fibrillation is likely to have recurrences.

We can see the bias in Lown's editorial by examining the last statement. Even in the early 1970s it was well documented and accepted by all cardiologists that nearly 30 percent of those who survive cardiac arrest as a result of an arrhythmia will be dead from the same condition sometime during the ensuing year. Clinical electrophysiology evolved in part as a response to this dismal statistic. But Lown apparently attempts to sweep under the rug carefully obtained clinical data.

Mirowski was stung by this rebuke in *Circulation*. It was painfully embarrassing to him that his first attempt to leave a personal medical legacy and save countless lives at the same time was so threatening to his profession. A bitter taste is the residue.

I'm not a psychologist and cannot analyze the violent reaction of others towards me and the implantable defibrillator, but I guess my colleagues had their territories firmly in place and we were trespassing. To put it plainly, I was attacked because in science, since time immemorial, new concepts are frequently not favorably received.

It would be humorous — if it weren't so ludicrous — that on the one side you have a few guys working in the basement of a community hospital in Baltimore, experimenting on dogs and not on patients, and on the other side you have an official journal of the American Heart Association publishing a three-page editorial in which distinguished cardiologists are making a special effort to eloquently prove that the implantable defibrillator could not and should not be built. The way I see it if somebody is proposing a stupid concept, the best thing to do is ignore him and if the concept is not valid it will die by itself. Obviously, those at *Circulation* didn't believe that I was proposing a stupid concept.

Mirowski and Mower responded to the *Circulation* editorial with a letter in the May 1973 issue:

> In contrast to Dr. Lown . . . we are aware of no effec-tive long-term antiarrhythmic regimen capable of reducing the prohibitive toll of sudden coronary deaths. . . .

And Mirowski and Mower added that the wariness and pes-simism directed toward the implantable defibrillator was "pre-mature," considering that the AICD was only in its experimental, prototype stage. They posited that it would be more appro-priate to suspend judgment of "this new way of approaching a major cause of mortality" until after clinical trials.

Unfortunately, Mirowski never got the last word in this de-bate. Dr. Lown responded with this "Author's Reply":

> No society, whatever its wealth, can adequately respond to all social needs. . . . We continue to be unpersuaded that . . . [this] costly electronic device provides a legiti-mate answer to the problem of sudden death justifying diversion of scarce social resources for its development.

The underlying message: the mainstream medical community will be the sole arbiter of what are acceptable clinical research and design efforts and of which projects deserve moral and financial support.

Mirowski's brief letter published in *Circulation* was one of the first statements that he was able to get in print concerning the implantable defibrillator. Most of his initial papers were rejected by the leading medical journals, which decide what to publish and what to turn down through a peer-review process usually weighted toward traditional medical ideas.

> We had a lot of difficulty publishing our first paper particularly. It was rejected on a systematic basis. One journal after another said it wasn't fit for its pages. It is

incredibly ironic that *Circulation* afforded so much space for attacking the implantable defibrillator and no space at all for our papers supporting it. I suspect that there were one or two reviewers who were specialists in the field of sudden death — but antagonistic to the implantable defibrillator — to whom our first papers were consistently referred. It was a no-win situation.

The resistance of the medical community to their project was a distraction, but Mirowski and Mower were steadfast in not letting themselves lose sight of their goals. What was even more disturbing, though, was a design impasse that Mirowski struggled with for months on end during the early 1970s.

The external defibrillator is a bulky device; it weighs about as much as a color television set. The reason for its size lies in its specifications and components. To deliver upwards of 300 joules instantaneously to revert an arrhythmia requires a massive bank of capacitors that occupies most of the space and volume of the external defibrillator. Batteries, which unlike capacitors can be miniaturized to power smaller electrical devices with an economy of scale, simply cannot output 300 joules consistently and repeatedly. So the problem that Mirowski faced was: how can the external defibrillator be miniaturized so that it is implantable in the body and still provide the needed power pack to revert an arrhythmia adequately in life-threatening situations?

Mirowski mulled over this quandary in pages and pages of equations and notes. He sought advice from engineers and biomechanics and electronics experts and applied it to his own knowledge of physiology and cardiology. Still the solution seemed distant and unreachable.

Suddenly, one afternoon, while Mirowski was making the rounds of patients, the answer came to him. As soon as Mower arrived at the Sinai basement lab that night, Mirowski said to him:

The solution is simple. If we cannot enter through the door, then let's enter through the window. If we cannot produce an implantable defibrillator capable of delivering 300 joules, then let's investigate whether we really need 300 joules to defibrillate the heart?

With that the constraints were removed from Mirowski's research. Facts started falling rapidly into place. For instance, during open heart surgery, surgeons frequently defibrillate a heart with only 20 or 30 joules. Moreover, a careful examination of the physiology of defibrillation in the electrophysiology lab turned up an intriguing fact: time and time again up to 90 percent of the 300 joules delivered to the closed chest is wasted in the tissues surrounding the heart; it dissipates before reaching the ventricles and atria.

This was encouraging data. It enabled us to conclude that a jolt targeted directly at the inner sanctum of the heart could be as small as 10 to 40 joules and still perform adequately as a deterrent to an arrhythmia. With heart arrhythmias you really don't need to deliver an atomic bomb. We can get by with a much simpler method of destruction — but only if it is a direct hit.

To ensure a direct hit, Mirowski designed a system of catheters and electrodes that attached directly to the heart. This meant that open heart surgery was required to embed the implantable defibrillator in the body — an option that Mirowski had hoped to avoid because of the attendant risks. But it also meant that tiny batteries powering a short, low-joule burst of energy could be used to spark the miniaturized AICD. In retrospect, Mirowski says, it was pure ignorance about electronics that was the difference between being stymied by and overcoming the obstacle of shrinking the defibrillator enough for implantation in the body.

Fortunately, I'm a clinician. If I were an engineer, I would have been convinced that I could never miniaturize the defibrillator, because I would still be focused on the problem of diminishing that large bank of capacitors.

Once the implantable defibrillator was miniaturized, the AICD was, at least in Mirowski's view, a fait accompli. Smooth sailing through a flood of naysayers marked the rest of the 1970s for Mirowski and Mower. In 1976, an implantable defibrillator was attached to the heart of a dog with chronic arrhythmias — and it reverted one failing canine heart rhythm after another. Finally, in 1980, the first human implant of the AICD was performed. With the success of this operation, the implantable defibrillator was approved for use in humans under experimental conditions, the initial step leading up to FDA approval of the device for general use five years later.

The implantable defibrillator is still only a last-resort device. Despite the fact that the electrophysiology community is itching to use it more often on patients with arrhythmias, it cannot. Subtle political pressures and powerful economic forces dictate against it. However, there is nothing less than a double standard at work here. Traditional cardiologists commonly recommend bypasses — still a dubious medical procedure in some groups of patients — as a first resort, but electrophysiologists are constrained from implanting AICDs — statistically more efficacious than arrhythmia drugs — unless pharmacological therapies have reached the very end of their long mentally and physically painful roads.

Thus for an arrhythmia victim to receive an implantable defibrillator he must have a history of at least one — and often two — episodes of severe ventricular tachycardia or ventricular fibrillation and there must be ironclad evidence of incomplete protection from an arrhythmia despite a long-term pharmacological regimen.

The major design weakness in the implantable defibrillator is the potential for false shocks, where an uncomfortable electrical discharge is delivered to the heart despite the fact that no arrhythmia is present. Though a false shock is an infrequent aberration, it happens often enough to concern Mirowski and other electrophysiologists and to precipitate a full-scale effort to root out this glitch.

A typical case of a false shock occurred at the Medical College of Wisconsin in Milwaukee last year, when 69-year-old Leonard C., who had had an AICD implanted in June 1984, felt a sudden painful twitch suffuse his chest while he was bending over to pick up a dropped coin. No ventricular tachycardia precipitated this apparent mutant discharge from the implantable defibrillator. Leonard C.'s physicians were at a loss to explain his symptoms and told him to notify them immediately if they troubled him again.

They did recur — and even more uncomfortably the second time. The following week, Leonard C. felt three sharp shocks in his heart during a brief period while leaning down to change his shoes. As before, he suffered no concomitant arrhythmia.

This time Leonard C. was admitted to the Milwaukee Hospital. Examination in the electrophysiology lab revealed that the implantable defibrillator was undersensing and oversensing at the same time — that is, during the false shocks it was misreading nonarrhythmic events as tachycardia and responding to them with a burst of energy; worse still, if a true arrhythmia had occurred, the AICD would have ignored it.

Leonard C. was taken to the operating room, where his chest was opened and the AICD's electrodes were evaluated wire by wire. Technicians discovered that the contact of one of the electrodes screwed into Leonard C.'s heart was intermittent because of two fractured wires. They were replaced and no sensing malfunctions have occurred since.

Leonard C.'s case is not typical by any means. In most patients the implantable defibrillator has been nearly foolproof, operating without failure. Further, it is expected that new models of the AICD will be enhanced with improved sensing componentry and a variety of programmable treatment options.

Having an AICD implanted is not an inexpensive proposition for a patient; it can cost up to fifty thousand dollars, including hospital, laboratory, and doctor bills. It should be noted, though, that this figure is a cumulative one and includes all medical costs leading up to the decision to implant an AICD — such as electrophysiological testing and the whole gamut of unsuccessful pharmacological treatments. Indeed, if the implantable defibrillator were prescribed as a first-choice clinical option, rather than an end-of-the-road procedure, the total price tag for the AICD would probably be in the range of thirty thousand dollars.

In most situations, health insurance covers at least a part of the cost of the implantable defibrillator. The federal government's Medicare program, for instance, which is usually slow to approve for reimbursement high-ticket items that are not the darlings of mainstream medicine, recently gave the nod of acceptance to the AICD, but termed the device "an investigational medical technique" in the process.

Using precisely chosen phrases, Dr. Enriqué Carter, director of the federal Office of Health Technology Assessment, which decides on the medical procedures and devices eligible for reimbursement by the Medicare bureaucracy, describes the decision to include the implantable defibrillator in the Medicare fold:

> In the instance of the implantable defibrillator we are dealing with a very grave, highly morbid, highly life-threatening condition of patients who are survivors of sudden death and have a probability of dying, and for whom other alternatives have failed. In those patients it is clearly necessary medical care, however investigational, because it prevents loss of life in a setting in which no alternative method exists by which to do that. So we have to allow technologies that might not yet be perfected into the marketplace as established medical care, or at least as necessary medical care, since they are available for life-saving purposes and no other alternatives exist.

This kind of skepticism is commonplace for Michel Mirowski, who has endured much sharper barbs during the past twenty years. Mirowski, though, now seems comfortable with what he has achieved, and is willing to let the future decide his place in medical history.

In the end the implantable defibrillator will be judged by one simple criterion: how well it accomplishes its goal of saving lives and giving years back to those who lost those years to begin with. If the implantable defibrillator saves lives, my side wins; if it doesn't, then they were right and I was wrong.

He winks; a shy grin crosses his face:

So far I have the edge, eh?

·15·

The Future

THE future for arrhythmia research is a bright one. Through the compelling argument of excellent results with patients who suffer from life-threatening arrhythmias, electrophysiologists are gaining broad acceptance in the cardiology community. Patients formerly left for dead by mainstream cardiologists are increasingly being referred to electrophysiologists, and in greater and greater numbers these patients are walking out of hospitals with their lives intact again.

But the very key to a successful future for electrophysiology lies in being able to identify and treat *before the arrhythmia occurs* those patients who will fall prey to a life-threatening arrhythmia. It's not enough to cure an arrhythmia after it happens; the vast majority of arrhythmia victims die well before they reach the hospital.

Says Jeremy Ruskin: "Realizing that in about half of all patients who die suddenly a lethal arrhythmia is the first manifestation of a heart problem, our most important challenge is to prevent the initial attack. The goal is to identify and treat those patients at highest risk for life-threatening arrhythmias without sacrificing larger numbers of patients to unnecessary therapy."

So far no such means exist, but there are hints that clinical investigative techniques for isolating those most susceptible to an arrhythmia are on the verge of being developed. Already, in one subgroup of patients — those who were victims of a heart attack — electrophysiologists are with increasing accuracy able to identify individuals at risk for a life-threatening arrhythmia. Dr. Thomas Bigger and his colleagues at Columbia-Presbyterian Medical Center did much of the ground-breaking research in this area. By combining information taken from patient medical histories with radioisotope scans of the heart — in which a small amount of radioactive material is injected into the body to detect, through its interaction with cardiac muscle and tissue, a diseased heart — a profile of the prearrhythmic patient has been discerned; in short, a model of the heart attack victim at risk for tachycardia or fibrillation has been constructed.

Bigger notes: "In our studies, 5 percent of the heart attack patients are in this high-risk group for arrhythmias. This represents as many as 50,000 patients each year who should receive more attention in follow-up studies and clinical trials to determine if we can reduce this incredible potential mortality rate. It would not be too aggressive to perform invasive electrophysiological diagnostic work on these patients, like attempting to stimulate the arrhythmia through pacing and then treating the arrhythmia if one is found. We could reclaim a lot of very ill heart attack patients by perfecting these models and using them as statistically sound diagnostic tools."

As for the rest of the population, it is hoped that improved electrocardiographs will enable even primary care physicians in Main Street office settings to identify those with a risk for life-threatening arrhythmias. The problem with current electrocardiographs is that when you "raise the volume" on them, in an attempt to make them more sensitive to the most subtle electrical aspects of the heart beat, the EKG becomes a cacophonous jumble, depicting without discrimination all of the noise in the chest.

But future generations of electrocardiographs will contain extremely advanced signal-processing capabilities, which will enable them "intelligently" to reorder the noise and electrical patterns emerging from the heart. These electrocardiographs will ignore and shrink certain irrelevant artifacts, while other important electrical signals of the heartbeat will be registered clearly. The result will be that this new brand of electrocardiograph will actually be able to detect currently indiscernible electrical disturbances in the heart and ignore the more typical noises and patterns that at present conceal these important signals from view.

"I have it clear in my mind — and if I can't live up to this, I'll eat my words — that between now and the year 2000 we will be able to identify most of the potential victims of sudden cardiac death before they experience a sustained ventricular arrhythmia," says Bigger. "I believe that we will be able to do this with considerable specificity so that patients who are not destined for sudden cardiac death are not inconvenienced by treatment and so the cost is reasonable. There are sensitive signals in the EKG sending us messages about the likelihood of future sudden cardiac death that will soon be readable by advanced signal-processing techniques. And when this technology is perfected, we could get to the point where we'll actually be willing to open a patient's chest and implant an automatic defibrillator. This research could save thousands of lives per year."

As for the implantable defibrillator that so many elecrophysiologists see as the ultimate treatment to prevent sudden cardiac death from arrhythmias, they, too, are in the process of being overhauled and redesigned. The next generation of implantable defibrillators will be able to be custom programmed for the individual needs of each patient. In the new devices, expected to be ready within a year, all settings will be adjustable, depending on the particular type of arrhythmia a person has. Dr.

Debra Echt, director of the electrophysiology laboratory at the Vanderbilt University School of Medicine in Nashville, Tennessee, describes the next round of implantable defibrillators as "nothing less than futuristic, compared to the primitive devices that are available today."

Essentially, we will be able to write a "prescription" for an individual patient based on the results of the testing we have done in the electrophysiology laboratory, which will tell the defibrillator exactly how to treat this patient's particular ventricular tachycardia.

For example, we will be able to program the defibrillator such that if the patient's tachycardia is at a rate of 145 beats per minute, the AICD would first deliver rapid pacing, rather than a shock, at a rate of 160 beats per minute to try to terminate the tachycardia, and it will perform this three times if necessary. After the third attempt, if the implantable defibrillator does not terminate the ventricular tachycardia through pacing, it would deliver a countershock of five joules. If the tachycardia gets faster, or turns into fibrillation, the defibrillator would then immediately deliver a countershock of 30 joules.

These new devices will also have a memory, so that when patients have received treatment by the device and return to our offices, we can noninvasively retrieve what the heart rhythm looked like at the time the device started its treatment. We can then determine what it was treating, whether it was effective, or if it was treating the right problem.

Meanwhile on another front, electrophysiological researchers are learning more and more about how the nervous system affects heart rhythms. Says Thomas Bigger: "We're getting to a point where we're understanding what the brain thinks and does about circulation and electrical connections in and around the heart, by analyzing patterns of heart rate or blood pressure oscillations. We are learning to decode noninvasively the signs that tell us about the balance in the autonomic nervous system and permit us to correct risky imbalances."

It has been suggested by some electrophysiologists that the lowered incidence of sudden cardiac death among heart attack patients who take beta-blocking drugs may be due to the way these drugs obstruct the sympathetic nervous system. The feeling is that perhaps, for patients at high risk for arrhythmias, drug therapies could be developed that alter the kinds of signals the brain sends out to precipitate electrical disturbances in the heart. This is currently extremely nascent research, but is considered an important avenue to follow by anti-arrhythmia strategists.

But beyond all of the clinical work to move electrophysiology into a future of greater achievements and successes, one uncompromising fact remains: in this country, sudden death is 85 percent to 95 percent a coronary heart disease problem. The most frequent predictor of life-threatening arrhythmias is damaged heart muscle. Obstructed blood circulation to the heart, blocked coronary arteries, cardiac scars resulting from a heart attack, and enlargement of cardiac cells commonly caused by severe high blood pressure impinge on the heart's electrical system and often, in time, transform normal heart rhythms into chaotic ones. By reducing the incidence of coronary heart disease, the chances of sudden cardiac death by arrhythmias is also greatly minimized.

Preventive medicine for heart disease, then, is a chief component for thwarting arrhythmias. Electrophysiologists emphasize that all physicians must become better at counseling their patients on the extreme importance of modifying and eliminating the elements of one's behavior and life-style that predispose a patient to cardiovascular disease from their day-to-day living. These risk factors are cigarette smoking, high blood pressure, indolence, excessive calories, negative psychosocial influences, alcohol consumption, and a diet rich in saturated fats and cholesterol.

Unfortunately, asking physicians to teach patients how to keep their hearts healthy through modifying risk factors is a major challenge. Studies of physician attitudes and aptitudes in cardiovascular preventive medicine have shown that, in the course of a ten-minute session with a cardiovascular patient, the way that most doctors deal with risk factor reduction is through glib oral advice and nothing more. A physician will commonly say to a patient, "You'd better ——— (fill in the blank with 'quit smoking'/'lose weight'/'cut down on salt,' etc.) or you're going to have a heart attack," and then drop the subject. For some patients, this scare tactic works extremely well, at least in the short term; for others, it falls on frightened but unheeding ears. Upon close inspection it's small wonder that many physicians are inept when it comes to advising their patients on the need to reduce risk factors and on the means to reduce them. A survey of the most frequently used cardiology textbooks show that an average of fewer than three pages are devoted to risk factors, risk factor reduction, and cardiovascular preventive medicine. However, to most cardiologists, who confront on a daily basis the ravages of atherosclerotic heart disease, and to electrophysiologists who constantly face the arrhythmias' deadly toll, preventive medicine is seen as paramount. "As important as learning to treat the disease is learning how to treat the nondiseased heart with tender, loving care," says Thomas Bigger.

The agenda, then, is set. Building upon five years of almost unparalleled clinical success, as well as the resistance and controversy that their research has engendered, electrophysiologists are finally beginning to make slow but steady progress toward a solution for arrhythmias. No one is promising a miracle overnight, but electrophysiologists are clearly taking the essential first steps toward some day defeating our most lethal disease.

·16·

Questions and Answers About Arrhythmias

What are the two types of life-threatening cardiac arrhythmias?

1)Ventricular tachycardia. A condition in which abnormal electrical impulses, which take over the pacing of the heart, originate from a site in one of the ventricles, far from the heart's normal pacemaker. With the heartbeat emanating from this aberrant source, often at a very rapid rate, the heart muscle may fail to fill and contract normally. Patients may experience anything from no symptoms to palpitations, weakness, and, sometimes dizziness or fainting. Ventricular tachycardia may be a precursor to ventricular fibrillation.

2)Ventricular fibrillation. This condition is related to ventricular tachycardia except that, instead of a single site in the ventricles delivering an abnormal electrical signal, multiple aberrant impulses course through the ventricles in a rapid and chaotic pattern. The heart contractions become so chaotic and ineffective that very little blood is pumped to the brain and the body and loss of consciousness occurs rapidly.

What are the symptoms of life-threatening cardiac arrhythmias?

The symptoms of ventricular tachycardia may range from minimal to severe and include: heart palpitations (a pounding in the chest) with or without varying degrees of lightheadedness, fainting, shortness of breath, sweating, dizziness, and blackouts. Typically, life-threatening cardiac arrhythmias are not painful, although in some cases they may provoke chest pressure or pain.

Ventricular tachycardia can go on for many hours, or cardiac arrest can be immediate. It is imperative that a person who experiences symptoms similar to those listed above and who feels clearly different from any way he or she has ever felt before seek medical attention, especially if the symptoms persist for more than a few minutes.

What is the initial out-of-hospital treatment for a person who suffers a cardiac arrhythmia attack?

If the person has arrhythmia symptoms but is not unconscious, call an ambulance and get him or her to the hospital immediately.

If the person is unconscious, call an ambulance, report a cardiac emergency — so that the rescue unit, if one is available in the area, is dispatched — and immediately initiate cardiopulmonary resuscitation. CPR is imperative, because the cardiovascular system of a person whose pulse and breathing are seriously impaired must be supported by cardiopulmonary resuscitation if brain damage and death are to be averted.

However, in the case of cardiac arrest as a result of a cardiac arrhythmia, CPR for an extended period of time cannot be the only treatment, if a good outcome is to occur. A rescue or EMT unit must defibrillate, or revert, the arrhythmia as quickly as possible — or the patient's chances of regaining consciousness and surviving cardiac arrest decline rapidly.

After surviving a life-threatening cardiac arrhythmia, what tests can a patient expect to receive in the hospital?

In-hospital tests that may be performed after a life-threatening arrhythmia include: electrocardiograms; chest X rays; cardiac scans or echocardiograms; exercise testing to monitor the heart's response to physical stress; Holter monitoring to record and analyze the heart rhythm for twenty-four hours or longer before and during the use of anti-arrhythmic drugs; heart catheterization to determine whether the coronary arteries which supply blood to the heart muscle are diseased and to define the extent to which the left ventricle, the main pumping chamber of the heart, is damaged; and electrophysiology studies to diagnose and help select treatment for the life-threatening arrhythmia.

What tests are used to develop a long-term strategy for treating a life-threatening arrhythmia?

The two most widely used tests in patients with life-threatening arrhythmias are Holter monitoring and electrophysiology studies. Holter monitoring involves the use of a tape-recording device to record the patient's heart rhythm for twenty-four hours or longer. These recordings are analyzed for the presence of abnormal rhythms, such as ventricular tachycardia; if frequent abnormalities are present, Holter monitoring is repeated while the patient receives an anti-arrhythmic drug. If the drug produces a favorable effect and eliminates or reduces the heart rhythm abnormalities that were present on the first recording, the patient may be treated with that drug on a long-term basis. Unfortunately, many patients (perhaps 50 percent or more) who have survived a life-threatening arrhythmia do not show sufficient abnormalities on a Holter monitor test to allow their physicians to use this technique to help develop a long-term treatment strategy. In these patients, electrophysiology studies are the most effective means of analyzing and selecting treatment strategies for life-threatening arrhythmias. Electrophysiology studies are also necessary in any patient in whom treatment with surgery, catheter ablation, or an implantable defibrillator device is being considered.

During the electrophysiology study, the patient lies on a padded table, above which is located a fluoroscope. One or more sterile catheters are inserted under local anesthesia into a vein and positioned inside the heart under X-ray guidance. The heart is then paced or stimulated electrically through one of the catheters, in order to reproduce the patient's arrhythmia under controlled conditions. After the arrhythmia has been induced and analyzed, it is stopped promptly by pacing the heart at a rapid rate (known as overdriving the tachycardia) or by delivering a shock across the chest with the patient asleep (known as cardioversion or defibrillation). The electrophysiology test is generally repeated in abbreviated form at other times to test the effects of anti-arrhythmic drugs on the patient's arrhythmia. In this way, the technique is used not only to diagnose the life-threatening arrhythmia but also to develop a long-term treatment strategy to prevent the arrhythmia from recurring.

What are the anti-arrhythmia treatments available to patients treated in cardiac arrhythmia centers?

There are four main categories of anti-arrhythmia treatments:

1.Drug Therapy. This is the first treatment technique used to thwart life-threatening arrhythmias. Anti-arrhythmia drugs are extremely fickle, though. There is no equation for deducing which anti-arrhythmia drug is the correct one for any individual patient. So, to test the efficacy and safety of anti-arrhythmic drugs before sending a patient home with a prescription, physicians in cardiac arrhythmic centers use trial and error, Holter monitor, and electrophysiology studies. First, a drug is administered to the patient for several days; then a Holter recording and/or an electrophysiology study is conducted on that patient, in which electrical stimulation of the heart is performed in an attempt to make the ventricular arrhythmia recur in the laboratory. If no sign of ventricular tachycardia or fibrillation appears, the drug is considered effective for the patient. But if a ventricular arrhythmia is induced, alternative medications are assessed in the laboratory until an adequate drug regimen is found. In numerous cases, no anti-arrhythmia drug is found that controls the patient's arrhythmia, or the anti-arrhythmia drug that stops the arrhythmia causes severe side effects. In these situations, the physician moves on to a different treatment strategy.

2.Catheter ablation. This is a treatment in which the patient's arrhythmia, mapped out during an electrophysiology study, is ablated by a targeted electrical shock delivered through a catheter. In essence, the area of cardiac muscle or tissue in which the arrhythmia resides is destroyed, so it can no longer conduct aberrant electrical signals. This technique is applicable to only a very small percentage of arrhythmia patients at the present time.

3.Arrhythmia surgery. Depending upon the type of arrhythmia and its cause, surgical therapy for life-threatening arrhythmias may involve either a coronary artery bypass operation or a special procedure directed at destroying the cardiac tissue that is responsible for the arrhythmia, or both. Destruction of sites within the heart that give rise to arrhythmias requires that these sites be localized or "mapped" by special electrophysiological techniques prior to and during the surgery. Once the responsible sites are localized, they may be ablated by any of a variety of techniques, including surgical excision, freezing with a cold instrument known as a cryoprobe, or vaporizing with a laser. Surgical therapy for cardiac arrhythmia is almost always an open heart procedure and is performed only at a limited number of specialized arrhythmia centers.

4.The automatic implantable cardioverter defibrillator. Also known by its acronym, AICD, this device consists of a pulse generator, which is implanted in a pocket of skin in the abdominal region, and three electrodes, which are either sutured to the ventricles of the heart or inserted into a vein and positioned inside the heart. When the pulse generator receives signals from the electrodes that ventricular tachycardia or ventricular fibrillation is occurring, a brief shock is delivered to restore the heart to its normal rhythm. In most cases this shock ends the arrhythmia. If it does not, the implantable defibrillator delivers as many as three additional shocks until the tachycardia or fibrillation is stilled. The AICD pulse generator is rectangular and weighs about two-thirds of a pound. In most instances a physician will not prescribe the AICD unless a patient has had at least one serious arrhythmic episode and all pharmacological alternatives have been exhausted.

What are sources of additional information about arrhythmias and electrophysiological treatments?

American Heart Association
National Center
7320 Greenville Avenue
Dallas, TX 75231

American College of Cardiology
9111 Old Georgetown Road
Bethesda, MD 20814

North American Society of Pacing and Electrophysiology
13 Eaton Court
Wellesley Hills, MA 02181

On the next pages is a partial list (supplied by the North American Society of Pacing and Electrophysiology) of clinical centers in the United States and Canada that can provide specialized care for patients with cardiac arrhythmias.

MIDDLE ATLANTIC

Dr. Thomas Guarnieri
Johns Hopkins Hospital
Baltimore, MD 21205

Dr. Enrico Veltri
Sinai Hospital
Baltimore, MD 21205

Dr. Sanjeev Saksena
Newark Beth Israel Medical Center
Newark, NJ 07112

Dr. Thomas Bigger
Columbia Presbyterian Hospital
630 West 168 Street
New York, NY 10032

Dr. John Fisher
Montefiore Hospital
Bronx, NY 10467

Dr. Anthony Gomes
Mt. Sinai Medical Center
New York, NY 10029

Dr. Leonard Horowitz
Philadelphia Heart Institute
Philadelphia, PA 19104

Dr. Mark Josephson
University of Pennsylvania Hospital
Philadelphia, PA 19104

Dr. Edward Platia
Cardiac Arrhythmia Center
Washington Hospital Center
Washington, DC 20010

MIDDLE WEST

Dr. Thomas Bump
University of Chicago
Chicago, IL 60637

Dr. David Wilber
Loyola University Medical Center
Maywood, IL 60153

Dr. Douglas Zipes
Krannert Institute of Cardiology
Indianapolis, IN 46202

Dr. Eric Prystowsky
St. Vincent Hospital
Indianapolis, IN 46202

Dr. Fred Morady
University of Michigan Hospital
Ann Arbor, MI 48109

Dr. David Benditt
University of Minnesota School of Medicine
Mayo Memorial Building
Minneapolis, MN 55455

Dr. Stephen Hammill
Mayo Clinic
Rochester, MN 55905

Dr. Rodolphe Ruffy
The Jewish Hospital
St. Louis, MO 63110

Dr. James Maloney
Cleveland Clinic
Cleveland, OH 44106

Dr. Albert Waldo
University Hospital of Cleveland/Case Western Reserve
Cleveland, OH 44106

Dr. Masood Akhtar
Mt. Sinai Hospital
University of Wisconsin
Milwaukee, WI 53201

NEW ENGLAND

Dr. Mark Estes III
New England Medical Center
Boston, MA 02111

Dr. Peter Friedman
Brigham and Women's Hospital
Boston, MA 02115

Dr. Jeremy Ruskin
Massachusetts General Hospital
Boston, MA 02114

NORTHWEST

Dr. Leon Greene
Harborview Hospital
Seattle, WA 98104

SOUTH

Dr. Vance Plumb
University of Alabama — Birmingham
Birmingham, AL 35294

SOUTHEAST

Dr. John Lister
Miami Heart Institute
Miami Beach, FL 33139

Dr. Robert Myerburg
University of Miami School of Medicine
Miami, FL 33101

Dr. John Gallager
Sanger Clinic
Charlotte, NC 28207

Dr. Paul Gillette
Medical University of South Carolina
Charleston, SC 29425

Dr. John DiMarco
University of Virginia School of Medicine
Charlottesville, VA 22908

SOUTHWEST

Dr. Frank Marcus
University of Arizona Health Science Center
Tucson, AR 85724

Dr. Christopher Wyndham
Presbyterian Hospital of Dallas
Dallas, TX 75231

WEST

Dr. Anil Bhandari
University of Southern California
Cardiology — 2025 Zonal Avenue
Los Angeles, CA 90033

Dr. David Cannom
Good Samaritan Hospital
Los Angeles, CA 90017

Dr. William Stevenson
University of California
Division of Cardiology
Los Angeles, CA 90024

Dr. Roger Winkle
Sequoia Hospital Medical Center
Redwood City, CA 94062

Dr. Melvin Scheinman
University of California Moffit Hospital
San Francisco, CA 94143

Dr. Ruey Sung
San Francisco General Hospital
San Francisco, CA 94110

Dr. Charles Swerdlow
Stanford University Medical Center
Stanford, CA 94305

Dr. Jay Mason
University of Utah Medical Center
Salt Lake City, UT 84132

CANADA

Dr. George Klein
The University of Western Ontario
London, Ontario, Canada NGA 5A5

Dr. Henry Duff
University of Calgary
Calgary, Alberta, Canada T2N 1N4

Index